Greenwood

Psychosomatic Gynecology

Psychosomatic Gynecology
A total approach to women's health problems

Lorraine Dennerstein
*First assistant, Department of Psychiatry,
University of Melbourne*

and

Eylard van Hall
*Professor and Chairman,
Department of Obstetrics and Gynecology,
University of Leiden*

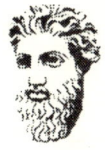

Parthenon Publishing
THE PARTHENON PUBLISHING GROUP LIMITED

Published in the UK by
The Parthenon Publishing Group Limited
Casterton Hall, Carnforth,
Lancs, LA6 2LA, England

Published in the USA by
The Parthenon Publishing Group Inc.
120 Mill Road,
Park Ridge,
New Jersey 07656, USA

Copyright © 1986; L. Dennerstein and E. van Hall

ISBN 1 85070 139 3

First published 1986

*No part of this book may be reproduced
in any form without permission from the
publishers except for the quotation of
brief passages for the purposes of review*

Typeset by Lonsdale Typesetting Services
Burton-in-Lonsdale, Carnforth, Lancashire

Printed and bound in Great Britain by
Butler & Tanner Ltd, Frome and London

For all our friends at the Department of Gynecology,
University of Leiden, whose enthusiasm and warmth
provided the impetus for this book

Contents

Preface		7
CHAPTER 1	The Psychosomatic Approach	9
CHAPTER 2	Therapy Techniques	21
CHAPTER 3	Sexual Problems	35
CHAPTER 4	Contraception	55
CHAPTER 5	Premenstrual Tension	73
CHAPTER 6	Infertility	87
CHAPTER 7	Chronic Pelvic Pain	105
CHAPTER 8	Hysterectomy	119
CHAPTER 9	Tubal Sterilization	139
CHAPTER 10	The Menopause	151
CHAPTER 11	Gynecological Cancer *(by Gerjanne Bos)*	167
Index		191

Preface

This is a book about a total approach to the problems of women's health. For many years, traditional gynecological practice has concentrated on the physical aspects of such disorders. Yet psycho-social factors are likely to be of especial significance in disorders of the genital tract as these organs are so intimately linked with inner concepts of femininity and sexuality. Both doctors and patients have become increasingly disillusioned with traditional approaches. Patients have formed consumer groups seeking more understanding and sharing of knowledge and a more active role in their own health and therapy. Gynecologists have sought to broaden their training in order to both meet patients' needs and improve therapeutic efficacy in the large number of disorders which have proved difficult to treat with traditional methods. Increasingly, expertise from the disciplines of psychiatry, psychology and social therapies have been utilized. How does the practising gynecologist incorporate such disparate approaches into everyday practice? When should the patient be referred elsewhere?

The intention of this book is to provide both a theoretical overview and a practical approach, enabling integration into clinical practice. The book is based on a series of seminars given whilst I was Boerhaave Professor of Psychosomatic Gynecology at the University of Leiden, and are the result of extensive collaboration with Eylard van Hall. We are both indebted to our colleague, Gerjanne Bos, who generously and readily contributed the chapter on psycho-social aspects of gynecological cancer, a topic not covered in the seminar series.

The first three chapters are largely descriptive, providing a theoretical understanding of diagnostic methods and therapeutic approaches. The remaining chapters cover selected topics, chosen as representative of the ways in which a broader understanding of biological, psychological and social factors leads to a more satisfactory therapy for both the woman and her doctor. It is hoped that the clinician will also apply this approach to other aspects of practice. A knowledge of the organic factors involved in gynecological disorders is presumed. The book is intended primarily for gynecologists, residents and medical students. Others interested in women's health may also find the book helpful.

Finally, the reader should note that the authors are aware that gynecologists and other therapists may be members of either sex. As it is cumbersome and distracting to write 'he/she', this book has used the accepted convention of English grammar. When the sex of a therapist is unknown the pronoun 'he' has been used. When 'he' appears in this generalized sense, please read 'she/he'.

Lorraine Dennerstein

Chapter 1

The Psychosomatic Approach

THE MEANING OF 'PSYCHOSOMATIC'

A great deal of controversy surrounds the term 'psychosomatic'. Some reserve such a term for psychogenically-induced disorders, others regard only a narrow group of illnesses as classically psychosomatic (e.g., asthma). For many it has become a derogatory expression. In community usage, psychosomatic is often interpreted as meaning 'neurotic', or 'all in the mind'. A historical perspective is useful in explaining these semantic differences.

The concept of mind-body unity is an ancient one. An Egyptian papyrus commented on the influence of the uterus on mental life. The 'melancholies of menstruation' were described by Greek physicians of the Hippocratic period. The term 'psychosomatic' was not introduced until the early part of the 19th century. Originally it was used to refer exclusively to mental symptoms such as phobias, obsessions and insomnia. The term was far from popular and was almost abandoned in the first part of this century. Ironically, this was a period in which theoretical models were being developed to explain mind-body links. Cannon and co-workers mapped the anatomical and chemical pathways connecting mental and somatic organs. Pavlov demonstrated that visceral somatic organs could learn to respond. Freudian theory developed, interpreting somatic symptoms as symbolic expressions of unconscious conflicts. The concept of target-organ vulnerability from infantile trauma was proposed. Medical opposition to Freudian theory continued with the lack of supportive evidence from prospective studies. Psychoanalytic therapy was often ineffective, especially when symptoms were not classically 'psychoneurotic'.

A major shift in theory took place during World War II, with the development of the specificity theories by workers such as Wolff, Dunbar and Alexander. Their theories discarded the notions of organic illness as being symbolic. Instead, specific personality patterns or emotions were linked to specific somatic diseases. During this period, Dunbar (1943) retrieved the term 'psychosomatic' and used it to describe both a somatic disease of psychic causation and an approach to the study of illness. Alexander *et al.* (1968) noted that certain kinds of conflict have affinity for certain organ systems. He related rage to the cardiovascular system, whereas conflicts involving dependency were directed to the gastro-intestinal tract. In his studies he focused on seven chronic diseases of 'unknown origin': peptic ulcer, bronchial asthma, rheumatoid arthritis, ulcerative colitis, essential hypertension, neurodermatitis, and thyrotoxicosis. These studies stimulated clinical research with many supportive findings. For example, duodenal ulcer sufferers could be predicted from psychological interview results of dependency conflicts (Weiner *et al.*, 1957).

Nevertheless, many of the psychological patterns could be observed in physically healthy individuals. Psychotherapy gave inconsistent results. With increasing scepticism of these narrow concepts, the definition of psychosomatic was broadened to include an approach to diagnosis and treatment that considered both psycho-social and organic factors. A scientific basis for this holistic approach gradually evolved, based on animal models, prospective studies and epidemiological evidence.

The new concept of psychosomatic is that of an understanding of the psychological processes in all disease and the manipulation of these factors to aid treatment. This concept is in keeping with current concepts of multiple etiological factors and causal networks in all disorders. The most widely used classificatory system in psychiatry (*The Diagnostic and Statistical Manual III* of the American Psychiatric Society) utilizes five axes which are to be considered in all presentations: clinical psychiatric syndrome; personality disorder; medical diagnosis; psycho-social stress; and social functioning. This approach eliminates the need for a simplistic formulation in which the clinician merely seeks to establish whether the disorder is organic or psychological. The intertwining of organic and psychological processes in both health and illness implies that all physical illnesses will affect mental well-being and similarly psychological illness often affects physical functioning. Psychological factors may exacerbate or diminish the course of an illness and affect the severity, discomfort and duration.

The object of the psychosomatic approach is thus to understand the patient, the illness and the response by consideration of all factors, biological, psychological and social. The method or manner in which this occurs is the doctor-patient relationship. This must allow the patient to communicate frankly and the doctor to perceive her messages, both overt and covert. Several factors are important in this process.

THE CONTEXT

It is expected that most women arriving at the gynecologist's office will experience some anxiety, especially if this is the first appointment. The anxiety is similar to that most people feel when confronted by a new setting, occupied by an authority figure. In addition, the woman attending the gynecologist is aware that she will have to reveal her most intimate self. Cultural and societal attitudes have influenced her expectations of the doctor and the consulting-room or hospital setting in which she will be seen. Further, her own socio-economic background, ethnicity, personality and intellectual skills will all influence her expectations and reaction to the therapeutic context. Certain aspects of the setting — if well considered — can help to allay anxiety and so help to establish the doctor-patient relationship.

The clinician should consider the arrangement of chairs, desk and examination couch. It is most important that the height should be the same for chairs for the doctor and the patient. Chairs should of course be as comfortable as possible. Placement of the chairs near a desk needs careful thought. If the desk is placed between the patient and the doctor it may serve as a barrier. By positioning the chair to one side of the desk the doctor has easy access to the desk without increasing the distance between doctor and patient. It is hoped that the doctor will not be writing continuously during the interview. To do so would prejudice his perception of the many non-verbal communications during the interview.

THE DOCTOR

There is some concern in the community that communication difficulties between doctors and patients may reflect real social differences, which may mean that the doctor perceives problems in a qualitatively different way from the patient. Until recently the gynecologist in most Western countries has been of a different gender, intellectual orientation and socio-economic background than the majority of patients. Such factors produce a social distance which the doctor then has to overcome in order to understand the patient's experience. Certain qualities in the doctor's manner may help to reduce social distance and form the basis for the therapeutic relationship.

Appearance

Acceptable hair and dress change with fashion. The patient's ability to relate to the doctor may be influenced by the doctor's appearance. The patient may question the maturity of the young doctor who accentuates his youth by wearing trendy or untidy clothes. If the doctor dresses in a provocative manner, an unwanted dimension may be added to the doctor-patient relationship. Such factors may undermine the doctor's status as a competent professional person. There is still debate about whether the doctor should wear a white coat. Those against this convention believe that the coat increases the distance between doctor and patient. Others note that this distance may be protective for the patient about to be examined gynecologically, who may well feel sexually threatened. Thus it may be necessary for a compromise to be reached between personal taste and the conventions of the clinical setting.

Availability

No-one is expected to be on call twenty-four hours a day. Nevertheless, the patient needs to know the arrangements for after hours care, especially for obstetrics. At a more personal level, availability implies that the clinician is concentrating on the patient and is not preoccupied with other problems. The patient may be less likely to divulge all her concerns if she is aware that the doctor is pressured for time.

Objectivity

In the working context of the therapeutic relationship, doctor and patient are equal participants. The patient supplies the subjective experience, whilst the doctor supplies an objectivity against which the patient's feelings, thoughts, behaviour, symptoms and signs can be evaluated.

Empathy

By this is meant the ability to understand the patient's feelings, without actually taking them on. To do so would imply a lack of objectivity and create a situation more akin to sympathy.

Acceptance

Respect for the patient as an individual is necessary in order to facilitate trust, the trust upon which the therapeutic alliance will be based. The therapist's acceptance of the patient's thoughts, feelings and symptoms as genuine are an important beginning to an exploration leading to understanding the patient. The doctor's acceptance may also be of therapeutic benefit for the patient, helping her to accept traumatic events of the past and other negative thoughts and feelings.

Non-judgmental attitude

The social system and expectations of the patient may differ from those of the doctor and are not of lesser value. A condescending or superior attitude of the doctor is likely to increase the social distance from the patient.

Confidentiality

Although this is often thought implicit by the doctor, it may be of benefit to discuss the concept with the patient. Adolescents may be worried that their parents will be informed of the interview. Another example is that of seeing a couple individually prior to marital or sexual counselling. There may be a great deal of concern as to how much information will be divulged to the partner.

Ethics

Related to confidentiality and trust is the concept that the therapist will respect the ethics of the doctor-patient relationship. This implies awareness of the potential influence the doctor may have on the patient and the intent to utilize this for the benefit of each individual patient. A special area of concern is that of sexuality. Eroticizing the relationship can only have harmful consequences for both doctor and patient. Both will have different expectations of a relationship in which they are of unequal status. Compromising situations and damaging experiences can be avoided, but only if the doctor remains in touch with his own and the patient's feelings. Thus the doctor aware of attraction to the patient may seek support from a colleague or refer the patient to another therapist who is able to maintain objectivity. Seductive behaviour by the patient may be dealt with by recognition of this and discussion with the patient.

Subjectivity

The clinician should remain in touch with his thoughts, feelings, value systems and motivations. By doing so, the evaluation of the patient will be greatly aided. Quite often the therapist's reaction to the patient is a mirror of how others perceive the patient and may be indicative of the patient's interpersonal relationships. Sometimes the doctor reacts in a certain way with a patient because of a triggering of emotions similar to those experienced earlier in life with a significant person. These feelings are sometimes called counter-transference. Always ask yourself how the patient made you feel and why.

THE PROCESS

For there to be a working relationship by which the interview process occurs satisfactorily the doctor must be a receptive listener and the patient must trust the doctor and be prepared to communicate.

The interview process requires both listening and observation. Although a great deal of information may be needed to have a full picture of the patient, this is not usually acquired in the format of a question and answer session. As Balint's work demonstrated, if you only ask questions you will only get answers!

A successful interview guides the patient through the history. The process is a dynamic one, during which the doctor is continually moving into the patient's position, withdrawing to ponder and perhaps seek clarification or comment, and then moving back into the patient's position and so on.

Content

Beginning the process

It is important to start where the patient is. This immediately establishes the doctor's interest in the patient as a unique individual. A question such as 'What brings you here?' may help to initiate the process. Unless the patient is otherwise known to the doctor, it is usually advisable to use the formal form of address of 'Mrs —' or 'Miss —'. This helps to establish that there will be boundaries to the session and the relationship. During the interview the doctor puts together, like a jigsaw, the symptoms of the patient, the relevant psychological, social and organic information and the observed information from physical examination and mental status. From this integrated material an understanding or formulation of the patient is produced which includes a diagnosis or explanation of the patient's complaints and has implications for therapy and prognosis. During the interview the following information should be sought:

Who is the patient?

Details of age, occupation, parity, social and ethnic background and religion help to define the patient and provide a broad background for the doctor from the expectations, knowledge and experiences which he associates with this demographic information.

What is the problem?

This is revealed by the patient's description of her complaints, their duration and severity, and associated factors such as menstrual history and other gynecological information.

Development

Gynecologists sometimes consider personal questions intrusive. Yet without an understanding of the environment in which the patient developed it is difficult to understand her responses now. By explaining to her that you are trying to understand her as a unique individual rather than as 'a case of', co-operation is usually secured. The following broad questions may be helpful: 'Tell me about your background — where were you born? What was your childhood like?' Of particular importance are knowledge of any early separations and losses, and any conflicts in the parents' relationships with each other or with the child. These factors may imply vulnerability in the patient to later losses, or difficulty in establishing close relationships. A general question, 'Did anything unpleasant happen in your childhood or adolescence?', sometimes frees the patient to describe experiences of rape, assault or incest which may have never been discussed before. Such experiences may contribute to gynecological or sexual disorders. When the patient has a current sexual problem, further information of the sexual development should be sought (see Chapter 3). Details of educational and occupational background assist the doctor later when he explains the illness to the patient.

Current environment

In order to understand the patient's current social context it is helpful to know where and how she is living and with whom (alone, partner, children, parents, others). Once again a general question such as 'Is everything satisfactory in your relationship and your sex life?' allows the patient to describe problem areas. Information about her relationship with her children (if any) is also relevant. Her current contraception should be noted.

It is also relevant to acquire some information about the patient in a wider social context. Does she have a social network, in particular are there close friends in whom she can confide or is this woman isolated? The social network has been shown to be of importance in protecting against the effect of life stress. Enquiries should be made about stressful events in the last year.

Personality

Ask the patient to describe how she sees herself as a person. If she feels she has changed and that this may be related to her presenting complaints, ask what she was like before the problems began. From her descriptions and your own observations, including awareness of how she makes *you* feel, a general overview about the personality of the patient is made. The presence of exaggerated traits such as obsessionality or histrionic behaviour are usually evident during the interview. The diagnosis of personality disorder implies that problems of behaviour have been present continuously from early in life and are severe enough to produce subjective distress or cause significant impairment in occupation or social functioning.

Coping strategies

By this is meant the habitual ways in which the patient deals with stress, pain, and conflict. Knowledge of these helps to predict reaction to stress, illness, and co-operation with any therapy. Coping strategies may be classified as follows:

Mature: This person is able to integrate her needs with those of others and with reality. Strategies include the use of altruism, humour, suppression, sublimation and anticipation.

Neurotic: The strategies used all alter feelings or instincts rather than dealing with them. Mechanisms used include intellectualization, repression, displacement, reaction formation, dissociation and denial.

Immature: This individual utilizes strategies to alter the perception of distress but often in socially unacceptable ways. Mechanisms include those of projection, fantasy, hypochondriasis, passive-aggressive behaviour and acting out.

Psychotic: Bizarre strategies are used by a patient out of touch with reality. Features include delusions, denial and hallucinations.

Vulnerabilities

During the interview the doctor should make some assessment of the patient's vulnerability to stress. The following factors may indicate risk and have prognostic implications:

1. Current history: lack of confiding relationships, children under the age of 6, significant life stress in the previous year, use of immature, neurotic or psychotic coping strategies.
2. Past history: early separations, loss of a parent before the age of 11, previous depression following a loss, past psychiatric history.
3. Hormonal: mood side-effects whilst taking the oral contraceptive pill, post-partum depression, premenstrual depression, menopausal problems (see Chapters 4, 5 and 10).
4. Family: psychiatric disorders amongst close relatives.

Fears

Every interview should include the opportunity for the patient to ventilate her fears and concerns. Questions such as 'What do you think is wrong?' may help the patient to express her thoughts. Remember that reassurance and advice are useless if you do not know what the *real* problem is.

Examination

Adequate physical examination is of course essential in order to determine the role of physical factors in the presenting complaint. The gynecological examination involves a special sort of intimacy. Not infrequently the patient will reveal further information during this. The posture adopted by the vaginistic woman is immediately apparent, as she retreats up the couch away from the gynecologist, her legs held tightly together. Sometimes during the examination the woman will start to describe a traumatic event such as an abortion. It is as though she believes that the gynecologist now knows all, having examined her.

During the interview the doctor has also been examining the patient's mental state. He has observed her appearance and behaviour, noted her speech and thought content and flow, perceived her mood state and observed any perceptual or memory distortions.

Investigations

Any further tests, psychological or physical, needed to aid diagnosis should be ordered without delay. Some doctors are concerned that investigations such as laboratory tests might focus the patient on the physical aspects of her illness. This is less likely to occur if the reasons for the test(s) are explained clearly and the patient is made aware of the multiplicity of factors involved in the illness.

Understanding — diagnosis

The doctor's task is then to integrate the various pieces of information into a meaningful whole. This involves consideration of the subjective and objective, the symptoms and signs, psychological, social and physical factors and the results of any tests. The result of this understanding is the 'diagnosis', an entity which implies knowledge of etiology, treatment and prognosis. This information must then be translated into a clear and concise explanation for the patient at a language level she can understand.

REFERENCES AND FURTHER READING

Alexander, F., French, T. M. and Pollock, G. M. (1968). *Psychosomatic Specificity. Experimental Studies and Results*. Chicago University Press, Chicago, Illinois

Balint, M. (1957). *The Doctor, His Patient and the Illness.* Pitman Medical Publishing, London

Dunbar, F. (1943). *Psychosomatic Diagnosis.* Hoeber, New York

Edelwich, J. and Brodsky, A. (1982). *Sexual Dilemmas for the Helping Professions.* Brunner/Mazel, New York

Engel, G. L. (1967). The concept of psychosomatic disorder. *J. Psychosomat. Res.*, **11**, 3–9

Gallon, R. L. (1982). *The Psychosomatic Approach to Illness.* Elsevier North Holland Inc., Amsterdam

Kalucy, R. S. (1979). Psychosomatic medicine: A review of the discipline. *Aust. NZ J. Psychiat.*, **13**, 85–101

Weiner, H., Thaler, M., Reiser, M. F. and Mirsky, I. A. (1957). Etiology of duodenal ulcer. Relaxation of specific psychological characteristics to rate of gastric secretion (serum pepsinogen). *Psychosomat. Med.*, **19**, 1–10

Wolff, H. G. (1950). Life stress and bodily disease — a formulation. In Wolff, H. G. (ed.) *Life Stress and Bodily Disease.* Williams and Wilkins, New York

Chapter 2

Therapy Techniques

INTRODUCTION

Many different forms of therapy are available to the clinician. Gynecologists are well trained in the use of physical therapies, such as surgery and medication. Most are familiar with the techniques of physiotherapy which have special application to obstetrics and gynecology, such as pelvic floor exercises and childbirth preparation techniques. This chapter will focus on the principles of the different forms of psychological therapies. It is not intended that the gynecologist should become an expert in all these therapies. Some of the techniques, such as certain behaviour therapy techniques, could be easily integrated into gynecological practice. Other techniques require a prolonged training and more time with each patient than the gynecologist may find practicable. It is useful for the clinician to have a working knowledge of the principles and applications of each of these therapies, so that he is aware of the range of techniques which are available.

PSYCHOTHERAPY

Psychotherapy refers to the relief of psychological distress and disability by psychological means and involves specially trained therapists utilizing an articulated therapy. The medium of healing is thus communication.

Success of all forms of psychotherapy depends more on the personal influence of the therapist than do medical and surgical procedures.

There are many different types of psychotherapy. From a historical standpoint all can be subsumed under two categories: the religio-magical and the empirical-scientific (Frank, 1977). The former have been present since the beginning of human culture and still have appeal to many, even in our advanced industrial societies. Religio-magical therapies are based on a philosophy of health as a harmony of forces within the individual and with those in the environment and the spirit world. Illness implies a disruption of these forces. The therapist's goal is to restore this harmony by the use of special rituals. Healing powers are attributed to supernatural sources usually linked to a religious system. During the healing process the patient may enter an altered state of consciousness, which may facilitate the therapy.

The empirical-scientific psychotherapies probably began with the work of Mesmer, who believed his therapy was the scientific application of animal magnetism. Following discreditation of his theory, empirical-scientific psychotherapies continued as hypnosis. Psychotherapy became popularized with the development of Freudian theory. Behaviour therapies developed from the experimental work of Pavlov and Skinner. The empirical-scientific therapies are all based on the view that entities relate to each other by cause and effect. Therapists base their success on scientifically based methods, rather than the supernatural.

The shared goal of all forms of psychotherapy is to reduce distress and thereby enable the individual to satisfy his or her needs. Despite the striking differences in the theories and techniques, there are a number of features common to all psychotherapies. These have been described by Frank (1972), whose work has helped to demystify this complex area and reduce the seemingly adversarial stances adopted by different schools of psychotherapy. Common features include:

1. An intense, emotionally charged, confiding relationship with a helpful person, often with the participation of a group.
2. A rationale which includes an explanation of the cause of the patient's distress and a method for relieving it.
3. Provision of new information concerning the nature and sources of the patient's problems and possible alternative ways of dealing with them.
4. Strengthening the patient's expectations of help through the personal qualities of the therapist, enhanced by his status in society and the setting in which he works.
5. Provision of success experiences which further heighten the patient's hopes and also enhance his sense of mastery, interpersonal competence or capability.
6. Facilitation of emotional arousal, which seems to be a prerequisite

Therapy Techniques

for attitudinal and behavioural changes.

In Western societies psychotherapy is generally reserved for those in whom psychological factors are contributing significantly to distress. Frank (1986) categorized those persons receiving psychotherapy into the following:

Psychotics: individuals whose symptoms may possibly have an organic basis. Psychotherapy here is predominantly supportive, helping the patient to recognize and deal effectively with life stresses.

Neurotics: individuals who suffer from faulty strategies for dealing with stress, either internal or external, presumably due to experiences early in life. These patients and those in the next category form the majority of those in psychotherapy.

Psychologically shaken individuals are those who are temporarily overwhelmed by current life stresses, such as bereavement. Relatively brief and superficial help usually restores the previous level of functioning. If this is deficient further therapy may be necessary following resolution of the crisis.

Unruly individuals are often brought by others who are distressed by their behaviour. Examples are antisocial personalities and addicts. Motivation for therapy is often lacking.

Discontented persons struggling with boredom or existential problems are an additional group who may receive psychotherapy in more affluent societies.

Professionals may undergo psychotherapy as part of their training. Some schools of psychotherapy require this as a prerequisite.

The patients most often referred by gynecologists will be those temporarily overwhelmed by a crisis, and those with poor coping strategies or neuroses. The particular type of psychotherapy which may be of most help varies with the individual. Some are best helped by a long-term psychotherapy, such as psychoanalysis, others by behavioural techniques. The principles of these different forms of psychotherapy are summarized below.

PSYCHOANALYSIS

This was the first systematic use of a psychological method to alleviate symptoms and modify aspects of personality. Psychoanalysis is based on the work of Sigmund Freud (1856–1939). Freud developed an elaborate theory of personality development which emphasized the importance of early life experiences and the central determining role played by sexual needs. His theory of mental functioning and behaviour was based on the concept that much of mental life was unconscious. Instincts and conflicts beyond conscious awareness were manifested in dreams. Unconscious mechanisms used to prevent the surfacing of this material into conscious awareness included projection, repression, intellectualization, denial, displacement and rationalization (see Price, 1978). Freud believed that unconscious conflict could give rise to anxiety which could generate symptoms. He was able to access the unconscious through dream recall, hypnosis and with the technique of free association, the patient's uninhibited verbalization of everything in his mind. In classical psychoanalysis the patient was seen for four or five sessions a week, each of which was fifty minutes long. To facilitate the process, a couch was used so that the patient could relax, with the analyst sitting out of eye contact. Interpretation was used to help the patient gain inner understanding or insight. Particular attention was given to the patient's relationship with the therapist (transference). Manifested in transference were the recapitulations of relationships to parental and significant figures earlier in life. Transference was positive or negative depending on the nature of the relationship. It was generally advised that the psychoanalytic psychotherapist should have a personal analysis as a basic preparation for therapeutic work. By tracing his own development he was then able to avoid the many problems arising out of counter-transference.

Psychoanalysis claims its greatest therapeutic usefulness for the neuroses and personality disorders. The most suitable patients are under 40 years of age, intelligent, motivated for change, and psychologically minded with capacity for introspective understanding. The time involved has meant that the application of psychoanalysis is limited. Modified forms of psychoanalytic treatment developed which incorporated Freud's basic concepts and those which recognized other dimensions to human behaviour.

INDIVIDUAL LONG-TERM PSYCHOTHERAPY

This once-weekly psychotherapy incorporates concepts from psychoanalysis from pioneers such as Jung, who emphasized the importance of self-fulfilment as a positive goal, and Adler, who emphasized the social dimension.

Challenges that psychotherapy was no more efficacious than spontaneous recovery (Eysenck, 1952) led to research in psychotherapy to identify the important therapeutic aspects and modifications to expedite therapy. Therapy length may vary between three and eighteen months. The two aims are those of symptom relief and personality change. Patient selection is similar to that for psychoanalysis. Contra-indications include those of paranoid traits, poor impulse control, a life-long attitude of pessimism and an impossible social situation such as an unresolvable marital or family problem. Aspects of therapy include those of a therapeutic contract with clearly defined goals, the use of free association, and the therapeutic strategies of clarification, linking, reflecting, interpretation and confrontation. Transference (feelings displaced onto the therapist from unconscious representation of people important to the patient in early childhood) and counter-transference (the attitudes that the therapist develops towards the patient reflecting feelings and attitudes to important persons in his life, past and present) remain important aspects of the therapy.

The following case illustrates the application of these techniques to psychosomatic gynecology.

Miss A was a 26 year-old infant nurse referred because of increasing depression following hysterectomy and bilateral salpingo-oophorectomy performed eight weeks previously. In addition to feelings of sadness and hopelessness, she had many of the accompanying manifestations of depression, such as early, middle and late insomnia, appetite loss, low interest and energy and somatic manifestations of anxiety. The operation had been performed for persistent ovarian cystic disease for which she had undergone several previous operations.

Assessment revealed that the patient was the middle child in a family of three children, had an ambivalent relationship to her mother by whom she felt rejected, a warmer relationship with her father and a development marked by hospitalizations and geographical separations from the family to treat her asthma. She had suffered from severe pain and menorrhagia since the onset of her periods at the age of 14. It was apparent that there were unresolved conflicts about sexuality and childbearing. These and the patient's constant illnesses had inhibited her social interactions. She was living alone in a small flat.

The major feature of her mental status was her depression. She was not actively suicidal and there were no delusions or hallucinations present. She reported considerable difficulty in obtaining help for her depression. Her gynecologist had reassured her and refused to refer her to a psychiatrist. She had returned to her general practitioner, who had made an urgent referral.

As she was significantly depressed, initial therapy focused on establishing a relationship, providing an explanation for her feelings and anti-depressant medication. As the depression lifted, a long-term psychotherapy was commenced. The goals were to help her to come to terms with her body, sexuality, and infertility, to resolve the relationship with her mother and to help Miss A to find fulfilment in her life.

She was seen once a week for eighteen months. She made a strong positive transference initially to the female therapist, which at times had erotic connotations. These were managed by interpretation and confrontation. During the therapy she projected her anger with the doctors who had 'mutilated' her onto the therapist. As the anger with doctors resolved, she began to focus on the disturbed relationships within her own family. At about this time her first niece was born. This highlighted her own infertility and increased her depression. As these feelings surfaced and were gradually accepted, Miss A was able to enjoy being an aunt. Her communication with both her parents increased and she learned more about the problems they had experienced during her development. Therapy helped her to understand their experiences and accept her parents. She began to become more involved in the community and joined a sporting club. Her concept of sexual identity remained somewhat confused. She established a homosexual relationship, but believed she was probably bisexual.

When she concluded therapy she was well adjusted mentally, both to the gynecological problems and to her social environment. She had developed considerable insight into her behaviour and mental life and was able to utilize this constructively herself. She has returned intermittently since, often to share a major stress in her life. She has dealt with these with a mature and optimistic approach.

SUPPORTIVE PSYCHOTHERAPY

Supportive psychotherapy is often wrongly assumed to include any sort of superficial counselling in which the patient is reassured or encouraged. The derivation of support is 'portare' — to carry. In supportive psychotherapy the therapist 'carries' the patient, helps to sustain her when she is unable to manage her life independently. The inability to cope may be temporary; for example, following a stressful situation such as a bereavement. The short-term crisis-intervention techniques used to help resolve such situations are discussed later. Some individuals are chronically disabled by personality, neurosis or psychosis and require longer-term support. The aims are to promote the patient's best psychological and social functioning, to restore her ability to manage her own life, to prevent any relapse or further deterioration, and to gradually transfer the source of support to family or friends, if possible. The treatment is reserved for those who do not have the personal resources and psychological mindedness to cope with a more intensive therapy. An example seen by the gynecologist is the middle-aged woman who suffers from continuous anxiety-depression and is unable to tolerate stress. She may constantly attend the doctor with a multiplicity of physical complaints. While unable to express her emotional distress, she communicates her distress somatically.

In this sort of therapy, the doctor's role is more directive and the therapeutic relationship is not as close or intense as in long-term psychotherapy. Therapeutic strategies include those of correction of faulty ideas upon which fears are based; explanation of symptoms, medication and other problems so as to provide the patient with a rational understanding; direct advice to assist with particular problems, aiming at developing the patient's skills for coping with such problems in the future; suggestions and encouragement; modification of the patient's environment; ventilation of the patient's emotions; and other therapies as needed. Pharmacotherapy may be needed or behaviour therapy techniques such as relaxation training. The most important problem for the doctor is that of undue patient dependency.

BEHAVIOURAL PSYCHOTHERAPY

This form of therapy utilizes learning theory, based on classical and operant conditioning models, as its theoretical framework.

Techniques for modifying behaviour antedate the experiments of Pavlov and Skinner. Pliny the Elder recorded elementary forms of aversion therapy for alcohol dependence. Conditioning techniques were used to treat enuresis by a 19th century pediatrician. Early this century psychologists began to apply some of the principles developed from laboratory findings. A major impetus to the use of behavioural techniques came from the work of Wolpe in the 1950s. He devised a form of treatment based on classical conditioning, which had wide application for the treatment of the neuroses. Systematic desensitization remained the single most important behavioural technique for the next two decades.

During this time an approach to individual treatment evolved, the behavioural analysis. This involved a detailed description of symptoms and behaviours and the circumstances in which these appeared or disappeared, increased or diminished. The guiding principle was that if abnormal overt behaviour persisted, it was being maintained either by responses to the patient of other people, or by factors within the patient. Techniques such as those of flooding and implosion, response prevention, modelling and social skills training developed. The main area for treatment focus was the observable behaviour. The client-therapist relationship was not unduly emphasized, nor was the client's early life history unless relevant to current symptom maintenance.

Critics of behaviour therapy were concerned that such stimulus-response approaches consider a peripheral relationship while ignoring central processing and the human within the problem. Cognitive processes were recognized as the essential link between emotional feelings and physical symptoms, leading to disturbances in behaviour and psychological well-being.

Cognitive-behavioural techniques were further developed by Beck, who used these strategies to treat depression (Beck et al., 1979).

Some of the behavioural techniques useful for psychosomatic obstetrics and gynecology are described below.

Relaxation therapy

This technique may be used by itself, to reduce anxiety or tension, or in combination with other techniques, for example as systematic desensitization.

Relaxation methods differ. Progressive muscular relaxation focuses on particular muscle groups. The patient is asked to tense and relax in turn different parts of her body. Usually the procedure begins with the lower limbs, comparing a tense foot on one side with the relaxed foot on the opposite side. Gradually the muscles of the legs, pelvis, abdomen, chest, upper limbs, neck, scalp and face are progressively contracted and relaxed. Breathing exercises may be used in conjunction with these muscular exercises. Once relaxation of the body has been achieved, the therapist helps the patient to achieve mental relaxation as well. Techniques include those of suggestion and imagery.

Other techniques used to achieve relaxation of the patient include hypnosis, yoga and transcendental meditation. Audiotapes made specifically for each patient may be helpful between therapy sessions.

Relaxation techniques are of great use in obstetric and gynecological practice. They are widely used as part of childbirth preparation programmes. A special application in gynecology is the woman who becomes anxious about gynecological examination and reacts with a vaginistic response. General relaxation and special vaginal exercises will enable her to be examined without discomfort. Relaxation procedures are often incorporated in sex therapy techniques (see Chapter 3).

Systematic desensitization

This technique is used to help reduce anxiety about specific situations. The patient and therapist develop a hierarchy of situations from the least feared to the most feared. Over a number of sessions, the relaxation response is associated with each situation that previously evoked anxiety. The patient is first relaxed and then a neutral scene is described. A scene from the hierarchy is next described, while the patient is asked to maintain her relaxation. Once relaxation has been achieved using imaginal techniques, the woman is asked to practise the situation in real life. An example is the use of systematic desensitization to treat non-consummation with vaginismus. The hierarchy may begin with looking at the genitals and progress to touching the external genitalia, insertion of the fingers into the vagina, tampon usage, allowing the partner to insert his fingers and then intercourse. It must be emphasized that such techniques are usually incorporated into a broader therapy which includes specific attention to the woman's thoughts and feelings, those of her partner and their relationship together.

Flooding

In this technique the patient is presented directly with the feared situation rather than this being approached gradually. This may be done either in imagination or in real life. The relaxation response is again paired with the feared situation. This technique has been used with success in the treatment of phobias.

Cognitive-behavioural therapy

This is based on the premise that the way we process or perceive information leads to behavioural change and emotions which may lead to, or exacerbate disorder. Cognitive-behavioural therapy involves two approaches. Firstly, it seeks to change the patient's methods of perceiving, classifying, and organizing events, their impacts and meanings.

Secondly, other behavioural techniques are utilized to change the long-established response patterns related to those events which may originate from both internal and external sources. The combination of the two approaches seems to supercede the effectiveness of either one in isolation.

An example is the application of these techniques in the treatment of premenstrual tension (Morse and Dennerstein, 1986). Women were invited to enter a group programme intended to strengthen their own resources for coping with menstrual cycle changes. A detailed behavioural analysis over one menstrual cycle was then prepared. Group sessions were conducted weekly for ten weeks. The cognitive restructuring component used a rational-emotive framework to dispute and reverse self-defeating cognitions, and a verbally mediated stress programme in which women learned to confront and overcome challenging events of both an internal and external nature. Behavioural techniques included relaxation exercises and assertiveness training. This approach achieved a further reduction in symptomatology over that achieved by hormonal usage alone.

MARITAL THERAPY

Social changes post-war have had profound effects on the expectations and behaviours of couples and families in many nations. The need for help often seems to have outstripped the resources available. Marital therapy may be based on psychoanalytic or behaviour therapy principles. The therapist utilizing psychoanalytic theory is aware that the way the couple relate to each other may reflect their relationships with parental figures during childhood. These disturbed relationships will become more evident during therapy. The therapist may become the target for transferences from both partners. In marital therapy the emphasis is on the couple's relationship rather than on that of the patient-therapist.

Behavioural strategies include those of operant conditioning and modelling. The therapist assesses both the areas of conflict and the areas of satisfaction in the relationship so that a hierarchy of needs for each partner may be developed. The principle is that both partners give to the other something wanted and receive something in return. Behavioural approaches thus focus directly on the problems, rather than on dynamic factors which may underlie these. It is well suited to couples in whom interpretation may mobilize more anxiety than can be coped with.

Dominian (1986) notes that there are five main relationships between a couple: physical, emotional, social, intellectual and spiritual. The therapist should try to determine the aspect(s) of relating that are causing difficulties. For example, if the problems are predominantly physical ones, sex therapy techniques may be utilized. Where sexual problems seem to reflect difficulties in the emotional relationship of the couple, therapy should be first directed at improving this.

Ideally, marital therapy is conducted with both partners together. The therapist's role is that of a facilitator and teacher. The aim is to produce change, so that the couple can perceive the nature of their marital problems and learn new modes of relating towards each other. By exaggerating the faulty patterns of communication, the therapist may make the couple aware of where the difficulties lie. In addition to modifying patterns of communication, the therapist may have to help the couple to sort out issues of power. Marital therapy may be carried out by one therapist or by two co-therapists. Couples may be treated in a group format. This approach enables each couple to recognize that their problems are not unique and to learn from the experiences of others.

Problems arising during the course of therapy include the failure of the spouse to attend, the labelling of one of the couple as 'the patient', which diverts attention from the relationship — the real patient, and increasing anxiety or depression in one partner, which may necessitate referral for individual help. There are three common patterns of outcome. One or both of the couple may not want a reconciliation. Only two or three sessions are usually necessary to sort this out. Alternatively, both may attend therapy and learn new methods of relating and the marriage may continue. Thirdly, the marriage may neither progress nor deteriorate, but continue as before. When no progress is evident the therapist should terminate therapy until the couple feel more prepared to work at the relationship.

CRISIS-INTERVENTION

This is a short-term therapy designed to help someone overwhelmed by stress. A crisis may be described as an obstacle to important life-goals, insurmountable using the customary methods of problem-solving. Caplan (1961) has highlighted four phases of crisis: phase 1, arousal and attempts at problem-solving; phase 2, increased tension leading to distress and disorganization. Arousal now hinders rather than promotes coping behaviour. The individual may be unable to sleep and becomes fatigued; phase 3, emergency resources, both internal and external, are mobilized and novel methods of coping are tried; phase 4, continuing failure to resolve the problem leads to a state of progressive deterioration, exhaustion and 'decompensation'. Help may be offered early in this sequence, when the individual may still be able to mobilize adaptive coping resources, or later, when intervention by others becomes a matter of necessity. The types of problem dealt with in crisis-therapy include those of loss, change in status or role, interpersonal problems and problems of choice between two or more alternatives.

When the therapist is able to intervene early, his role is that of a facilitator. Thus, in the setting of an empathic relationship the patient is encouraged to communicate her feelings, to understand the meaning of the situation by identifying and defining the problem, to find alternative methods of coping with the problem and to rehearse these in turn so as to be aware of the implications. Although the aim is to help the patient to find a solution, on occasions it is justifiable to give expert advice. Psychotropic drugs are sometimes necessary, for example to improve a patient's sleep. If assessment reveals that the patient is unable to carry on, more intensive intervention is called for. This may involve the transfer of the patient's usual obligations to others, removal of the patient from a stressful environment, lowering of arousal and distress by warm, empathic discussions with the patient and, if necessary, by medication, and by reinforcement of appropriate communications by the patient. Once the shocked state has subsided, the crisis counselling techniques described above can be utilized.

HYPNOSIS

Hypnosis may be defined as an altered state of consciousness characterized by sensory, motor and cognitive phenomena. These phenomena include heightened suggestibility, failure of repression, trance logic, age regression, amnesia, time distortion, analgesia, anesthesia, and catalepsy. There are many misconceptions about hypnosis, such as the power of the hypnotist to work miracles or that only the gullible or the hysteric is hypnotizable. Research has found no relationship between hynotizability and personality, intelligence or sex. The majority of people can be hypnotized. The measurement of hypnotic susceptibility results in a normal distribution curve, with a group of people who are excellent subjects, another who are non-hypnotizable, and the majority falling in-between.

Hypnosis may be used as an aid to other psychotherapies or for the benefits produced by hypnotic phenomena, for example to relieve pain. Incorporation of hypnosis into behavioural therapy produces a deeper state of relaxation and increases visual imagery, and the increased suggestibility may be utilized therapeutically. Hypnosis may catalyze psychoanalytic-based therapies by rapidly increasing transference, overcoming repression, and increasing suggestibility. The therapist utilizing hypnosis needs training both in hypnotic techniques and in the psychotherapy in which the technique is to be incorporated. The latter may be limited when hypnosis is utilized for its phenomena, as in preparation for childbirth. In this example hypnosis may be used individually or in groups. The aim is to reduce anxiety and pain. Procedures include those of relaxation, imagery, labour rehearsal, and analgesia control. Post-hypnotic suggestions may be used to facilitate time distortion and amnesia, when the patient desires this. Other examples of the use of hypnosis in obstetrics and gynecology are the treatment of hyperemesis gravidarum, prevention of premature labour, for relaxation during breast feeding, and in conjunction with sex therapy techniques.

CONCLUSION

A number of different forms of psychological therapies are available which may be of help to the gynecologist. His role is firstly to identify the part psychological and social factors may be playing in the illness. Next a decision must be made about whether psychological techniques should be incorporated into the therapy. These techniques may be utilized by the gynecologist, or the patient may be referred to another therapist. Some psychiatrists and psychologists use only one type of therapy, adhering strictly to one frame of reference. Others adopt a more eclectic viewpoint in which they use the therapy which is appropriate to the individual at the time of presentation. It is helpful for the doctor to have some knowledge of the therapeutic stance of the psychiatrists and psychologists to whom he refers patients.

Many of the therapy techniques described in this chapter are suitable for use by gynecologists. Particularly suitable are the techniques of supportive psychotherapy and behaviour therapy. In utilizing such techniques the gynecologist and the patient need to re-examine their orientation and expectations of therapy. The responsibility for change is the woman's. Both doctor and patient must be active in such therapies. This represents quite a shift from the traditional somatic gynecology model in which the doctor is active in prescribing treatments and carrying out surgery and the patient is passive and powerless. An important component in the successful use of psychotherapies is the patient's motivation for change. It should be remembered that this is a dynamic and changing quality, not a stable trait. It is undoubtedly increased by personal distress. In assessing motivation the therapist needs to assess the relationship with the patient and that between the patient and her personal and general environment.

REFERENCES AND FURTHER READING

Beck, A. T., Rush, A. J., Shaw, B. F. and Emery, G. (1979). *Cognitive Therapy for Depression*. Guilford, New York

Bloch, S. (1986). *An Introduction to the Psychotherapies*, 2nd edn. Oxford University Press, Oxford

Caplan, G. (1961). *An Approach to Community Mental Health*. Tavistock, London

Dominion, J. (1986). Marital therapy. In Bloch, S. (ed.) *An Introduction to the Psychotherapies*, pp 149–71. Oxford University Press, Oxford

Eysenck, H. J. (1952). The effects of psychotherapy: an evaluation. *J. Consulting Psychol.*, **16**, 319–24

Frank, J. (1972). Common features of psychotherapy. *Aust. NZ J. Psychiat.*, **6**, 34–40

Frank, J. (1977). The two faces of psychotherapy. *J. Nerv. Ment. Dis.*, **164**, 3–7

Frank, J. (1986). What is psychotherapy? In Bloch, S. (ed.) *An Introduction to the Psychotherapies*, pp 1–23. Oxford University Press, Oxford

Morse, C. A. and Dennerstein, L. (1986). Cognitive perspectives of premenstrual tension. In Dennerstein, L. and Fraser, I. (eds) *Hormones and Behaviour*, pp 197–203. Excerpta Medica, Amsterdam

Price, R. H. (1978). *Abnormal Behaviour in Perspectives in Conflict*, 2nd edn. Holt Rhinehart & Winston, New York

Wolpe, J. (1958). *Psychotherapy by Reciprocal Inhibition*. Stanford University Press, Stanford

Chapter 3

Sexual Problems

INTRODUCTION

The last two decades have seen huge changes occur in attitudes, knowledge and expectations of sexuality and sex roles. Many factors have played a part in producing changes. These include social movements, the popularity of psychological viewpoints of sex as a central moving force in life, the availability of a range of effective contraceptive methods and the publication of a number of research findings into sexual behaviour.

Kinsey's systematically documented studies forced society to acknowledge the disparity between its view of how people 'ought to behave sexually' and how they did behave. Contemporary society re-evaluated its expectations of sexual behaviour from the image of sexuality described. Masters and Johnson subsequently elucidated the physiology of sexual response using direct observation and measurement in a laboratory setting. Medical undergraduates and postgraduates now have access to human sexuality courses. The behavioural techniques introduced by Masters and Johnson (1970) for treatment of sexual dysfunction have evolved into sex therapy techniques, now widely available in most Western countries.

The demand for knowledge of sexuality has been reflected in the world-wide success of many books for the lay public. Women's action groups have also fostered changes in both general and sexual expectations of women. Undoubtedly the mass media have played an important part in changing attitudes.

The liberalization of discussion of sexuality combined with the changing expectations of both men and women are at least partly responsible for the rapid upsurge of consultations on sexual concerns observed by both general practitioners and specialists.

Sexual concerns are of two types, those related to unrealistic expectations of sexual behaviour and those reflecting sexual dysfunction.

UNREALISTIC EXPECTATIONS

While public knowledge of sexual behaviour is increasing, it is far from adequate. Lack of knowledge and/or misinformation often result in unrealistic expectations. In the clinical setting unrealistic expectations of performance abound.

Concerns about orgasm often reflect misinformation. The novelist's licence to portray orgasm as a feeling of 'waves roaring in the ears' and other similar romanticized descriptions have resulted in many women being unaware of, or even disappointed in orgasm. Some women present with the complaint that orgasm is only reached during sexual foreplay with the partner and not during intercourse. Both the woman and her partner often feel they are 'missing out' and that this experience is not a proper orgasm. These commonly expressed views are a remnant of the Freudian theory that an 'immature clitoral orgasm' is transferred in the mature woman to a vaginally felt orgasm. Needless to say, lengthy analytic therapy has usually failed to effect a transfer. Masters' and Johnson's investigations have shown that there is only one orgasmic process, which may be elicited by different stimuli. Expectations that orgasm should occur only during the act of sexual intercourse are unrealistic.

Many people remain unaware of the changes in sexual functioning to be expected with age. Studies of sexual response in the elderly suggest that arousal takes longer for males and females. More direct physical stimulation may be required than was needed earlier in life to effect adequate arousal. Other age-related changes that may provoke anxiety include lengthening of the male refractory period and decrease in ejaculatory frequency.

Provided physical health remains satisfactory, adequate sexual response often continues into the seventh and eighth decades. Lack of knowledge of age-related sexual changes combined with the commonly held myth that sexual behaviour terminates in middle age are responsible for much unnecessary suffering. An example is the middle-aged male who fears he is 'over the hill' because he no longer readily achieves an erection on merely looking at his partner.

PSYCHOSEXUAL DYSFUNCTION

Approaches to understanding sexual dysfunction have moved this century from the psychoanalytic viewpoints of Freud to the physiological investigations of Masters and Johnson (1966). In their subsequent descriptions of sexual inadequacy in 1970, Masters and Johnson identified two types of dysfunction in women — orgasmic dysfunction and vaginismus. Kaplan (1979) later recognized the importance of cognitive factors, extending her biphasic model to a triphasic one — disorders of desire, arousal or orgasm. In understanding the interrelationship between cognitive factors and potency the model proposed by Davidsen et al., 1982) is a useful one (Figure 1). He proposed the term 'libido' to cover the sum of all cognitive processes including sexual drive, attitudes and feelings. 'Potency' is used to denote those behaviours associated with sexual activity such as arousal (erection or vaginal lubrication) and orgasm or ejaculation. The important feedback between libido and potency is identified. In the sexually healthy, positive attitudes, feelings and drive arouse or reinforce potency. In the sexually dysfunctional, negative emotions such as fear, anxiety or anger are inhibitors of potency. Organic factors may act at any level affecting potency by peripheral effects on the neurological, vascular or genital organs or centrally by affecting libido.

A major shift in sex therapy this decade has been the increased recognition of the importance of cognitive factors (the patient's own internal dialogue with him/herself), leading to the combination of cognitive restructuring techniques with the behaviourally-based sex therapy techniques. Thus resistances can be explored, attitudes changed and

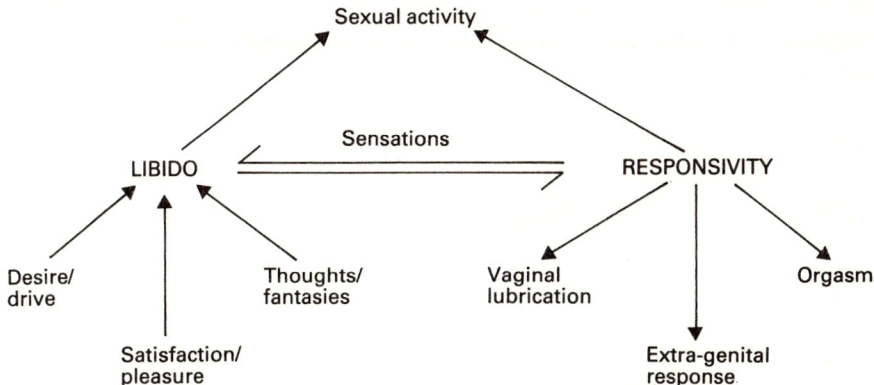

Figure 1   Components of sexuality. (Adapted from Davidsen et al., 1982)

coping techniques developed. Negative attitudes often reflect interpersonal conflict. The importance of assessing the relationship cannot be underestimated. Another major shift has been the increased recognition of the importance of organic factors in causing sexual dysfunction. Awareness of the role of hormones in both male and female sexuality has developed. Circulatory problems as causes of erectile problems in men are receiving increasing attention. The number of men presenting to sexual counselling clinics has increased, perhaps reflecting changed community stereotypes.

Types of sexual dysfunction

It is obviously preferable to specify the exact type(s) of complaint and the time duration rather than to resort to the use of ambiguous terms. As male and female sexual response are physiologically analogous, similarities are also to be found in the types of concerns expressed. These are briefly summarized in Table 1. As well as of the specific concerns listed, it is not uncommon for women to complain of general displeasure with secretion, smell or mechanics of sexual intercourse.

More than one type of concern may be present. A woman may complain of pain during intercourse, failure of vaginal lubrication and gradual loss of sexual interest.

Psychosexual dysfunction may be a primary phenomenon present in most sexual encounters experienced by the patient. Alternatively, and more commonly, the problem may have arisen after previously satisfactory sexual functioning. By the time consultation is sought there is usually considerable anxiety associated with the sexual situation. Any

Table 1 Sexual dysfunction: common presenting symptoms

Sexual response phase	Male	Female
Arousal	Inadequate sexual desire Difficulty achieving erection	Inadequate sexual desire Lack of vaginal lubrication Pain
Penetration	Failure to maintain erection	Non-consummation Pain
Orgasm	Ejaculating too quickly Failure to ejaculate	Failure to achieve orgasm

anxiety will delay or inhibit sexual arousal. As anxiety is experienced as an unpleasant emotion, sexual activity which results in an uncomfortable level of anxiety will tend to be avoided. Anxiety about sexual failure will lead to further failures and eventual avoidance of sexual behaviour.

ETIOLOGY OF PSYCHOSEXUAL DYSFUNCTION

Modern viewpoints recognize that there are multiple causes of sexual dysfunction, with remote and immediate causes existing side by side in dynamic equilibrium. The earlier approach of the Freudian theorists was that sexual dysfunction represented a manifestation of serious underlying unconscious conflicts often resulting from failure of psychosexual development in childhood. The behaviourists focused instead on the sexual symptoms presented. Rather than conflicts arising in the remote past, immediate causes were ascribed for symptom perpetuation. These included expectations of failure, demands for performance, fears of rejection and humiliation and poor communication with the partner.

For simplicity, etiological factors may be divided into three major groups. These are summarized in Table 2. It should be emphasized that causes from each group may be present simultaneously and that therapy techniques must be necessarily individualized for each couple.

Table 2 Major factors in psychosexual dysfunction

Symptomatic: related to some current cause
Interpersonal
Organic
Psychiatric
Alcohol and drug abuse
Iatrogenic

Learned: the stressful situation(s) no longer present, the behaviour continues in a learned manner
Family
Religious
Early and unpleasant sexual experiences
Gynecological disorders

Intrapsychic conflict: a manifestation of 'unconscious conflicts' between the desire to have sex and the fear of doing so
Failure of adequate psychosexual development
Restrictive childrearing
Religious influences

Symptomatic

The dysfunction is related to some *current* cause, which may include family, social, interpersonal, occupational, physical or psychiatric illness.

Interpersonal

Marital discord may be defined as a lack of harmony between the couple. The most common complaints of couples seeking marital counselling include constant arguments, non-, mis- or malcommunication, unfulfilled emotional needs, sexual dissatisfactions, financial disagreements, in-law trouble, infidelity, conflicts about children, domineering and suspicious partners. These complaints may be symptomatic of deeper disappointments and frustrations and are not necessarily the basic factors causing marital disharmony. Although sexual dissatisfaction may lead to marital disharmony, interpersonal problems in themselves are a major cause of sexual dysfunction. When one member of the couple has decided not to continue with the relationship this is sometimes evidenced in sexual avoidance and dysfunction.

An analysis of all patients referred with sexual dysfunction over a twelve-month period found that in one-third the sexual dysfunction reflected other problems in the couples' relationships. Interpersonal problems were the largest single cause of sexual dysfunction among the patients seen.

A common euphemism for sexual intercourse is the term 'making love'. The quality of the sexual encounter alters when loving feelings are not present. It is expected that when general communication is faulty and anger and conflict are present, sexual communication would also be poor.

Organic

Organic causes affecting sexual functioning may be general or local. General physical disorders may fall into one or more of the following conditions: systemic disorders such as infections, hematological diseases, malnutrition. Coronary or pulmonary insufficiency and metabolic disorders, such as those associated with hepatic or renal disease, may present with sexual problems. Endocrine disorders such as myxoedema or ovarian failure at menopause and genetic disorders such as Klinefelter's syndrome are also found. Vascular disorders affecting either major arteries or small penile blood vessels, and the neurological disorders such as multiple sclerosis, peripheral neuropathies and Parkinsonism are other causes. Post-traumatic conditions such as spinal cord transection may also affect sexual behaviour.

Multiple sclerosis and diabetes mellitus are examples of diseases affecting many parts of the body which may interfere with sexual functioning by associated neuropathy. Some general diseases or injuries interfere with sexual functioning not by their direct effects on body physiology but by their psychological significance to the individual concerned. An example is the sexual dysfunction following myocardial infarction. Some investigators have found that in one-half of these patients sexual intercourse decreased or ceased altogether in the twelve months following discharge from hospital. In many cases this was related to fears that sexual intercourse was too strenuous an activity and might precipitate another coronary attack.

Local organic causes of sexual dysfunction include congenital and acquired disorders of the genital area. Physical deformity resulting from congenital malformations in the genital area can often be improved with surgery. The psychological implications of the abnormality to the sexual identity of the person concerned may result in considerable psychological impairment unless there is early psychiatric intervention.

Any painful lesion in the female pelvic or genital area may result in pain with intercourse (dyspareunia), which will in time lead to loss of desire for sexual intercourse. Endometriosis, chronic pelvic inflammation and vaginitis are examples of organic causes of dyspareunia. Painful lesions of the penis or scrotum may similarly impair male potency.

Psychiatric

Sexual dysfunction sometimes occurs secondarily to other psychological illnesses such as anxiety states and depression. It is important to differentiate anxiety and depression which occur as a consequence of sexual dysfunction from anxiety states and depressive illness which pre-existed and caused the sexual concern. Usually mild anxiety and depression occurring secondarily to continued sexual failure respond rapidly to therapy of the sexual problem. Where an anxiety state or depressive illness pre-existed, clinical management should be directed at these conditions rather than at the sexual concern presented. Schizophrenia may be associated with pan-sexual disturbances. These include delusions of sexual identity or genital alteration and hyper- or hyposexuality.

Other sexual disorders arising in schizophrenia may reflect the quality of the relationship with the partner. When a general sexual dysfunction such as premature ejaculation occurs in a patient suffering from schizophrenia, the illness is not the underlying cause of the dysfunction. Specific therapy of sexual concerns in a patient suffering from schizophrenia is thought inadvisable in the acute phase of the illness. After the person becomes relatively stable mentally, specific therapy of the sexual dysfunction may be considered concomitantly.

Alcohol and drug abuse

Drug and alcohol users claim that small doses of alcohol or amphetamines, or the use of cocaine or marihuana, increase desire and enjoyment of sex and lower inhibitions. Central nervous system depressant-type drugs such as barbiturates, methaqualone, heroin and large amounts of alcohol decrease sexual activity. Large doses of amphetamines also have this effect.

Chronic alcoholism frequently impairs sexual response. This may reflect the neurological and hepatic damage and the general debilitating effects of alcohol. Men often first experience difficulty in achieving an erection after excessive alcohol intake. This may particularly occur in the older male. Anxiety about the sexual failure, combined with other stresses, which may have initiated the alcohol abuse, may perpetuate this problem.

Iatrogenic

Iatrogenic causes usually refer to problems resulting from therapies instituted by medical practitioners' suggestions.

Suggestion: The term 'iatrogenic' was originally applied to disorders induced in the patient by auto-suggestion based on the doctor's examination, manner, or discussion. Certainly, many concerns have as their origin ill-considered words stated by the doctor. It is not unusual for a doctor to comment, during the course of a gynecological examination, on some minor abnormality such as cervical erosion, cervical dysplasia, prolapse, retroverted uterus and bulky uterus.

While these terms may not imply major pathology to the doctor using them, they may result in considerable distress for many women. If the doctor requests more frequent follow-up smear tests because of cervical dysplasia it is likely that the woman, not understanding the natural course of this disease, will infer that something is very wrong inside her vagina. The woman who is told that her womb is 'bulky' instead of 'normal size for a woman who has borne children' may needlessly worry whether it is a 'growth' that is responsible. While the doctor is aware that retroversion of the uterus is a common variant, being present in one-third of women, his patient may wonder what harm will follow having a uterus in such an abnormal position that it caused comment by the doctor. Anxiety that all is not as it should be in the genitalia may lead women to fear that sexual activity may provoke further damage. Loss of desire for sex, difficulty in becoming aroused, dyspareunia and avoidance of sexual encounters may result from anxiety needlessly provoked by the physician.

Medications: Certain prescribed drugs may affect sexual behaviour by central or peripheral effects. Dopamine receptor blockers, such as haloperidol and phenothiazines, and depletors of dopamine, such as reserpine, interfere with the central control of sexual behaviour.

Peripheral effects of drugs on sexual behaviour reflect differential effects on autonomic nervous system components. Drugs which cause ejaculatory failure often interfere with sympathetic functioning. These include the alpha-adrenoreceptor blocker phenoxybenzamine, the adrenergic neurone blocking agents, guanethidine and reserpine, as well as ganglion blocking agents. Their use may result in retrograde ejaculation, or absence of emission and orgasm. The highest incidence of reported sexual side-effects is related to guanethidine, and there is some indication that this effect may persist long after therapy because of a selective depletion of noradrenaline stores in the internal genitalia. Reports of impotence with such drugs may reflect central effects. Ganglion blocking drugs affect both ejaculation and erection, reflecting their action on both divisions of the autonomic nervous system. Muscarinic blocking drugs such as the tricyclics, and the monoamine oxidase inhibitors also interfere with penile erection.

The oral contraceptive pill has been reported to cause sexual side-effects. The pharmacological and psychological or symbolic effects of contraceptive pill-taking are discussed further in Chapter 4.

Surgery: Surgery may result in sexual dysfunction by direct physical interference. Any extensive pelvic surgery which is likely to damage the nerve supply of the genitalia may result in sexual dysfunction (example: rectal resection). Local surgery involving the genitalia may also lead to sexual dysfunction. Prostatectomy not infrequently damages the nervous supply of the penis, with consequent failure to achieve erection in subsequent sexual encounters.

Episiotomy, obstetrical tears and other operative gynecological procedures may result in painful scars, a patulous or contracted introitus, a shortened vagina and damage to the sensory innervation of the vulva. The consequence may be failure of vaginal lubrication and dyspareunia.

Other surgery may interfere with sexual response because of psychosocial effects. Psychological reactions to surgery will depend on: the premorbid personality of the individual, current interpersonal relationships, the patient's emotional responses to the surgeon and the actual meaning of the operation *per se*. This includes the threat of danger, the amount of suffering to be expected, the chances of cure and the real and symbolic significance of the diseased organ. For example, after surgery resulting in a colostomy, even when nervous innervation of the genitalia remains intact, the effects on body perception and/or aesthetic aspects may result in withdrawal from sexual relationships.

Breast resection also is an operation which often has a devastating effect on body image. Breasts are revered in our society as a symbol of feminine sexuality. Loss of one or both breasts is a very stressful experience, especially as this disfiguring operation is made necessary by the spectre of cancer. Surprisingly few women are given counselling before or after this distressing operation. At least half the women interviewed in one series indicated that their doctor was not available to answer questions. Not surprisingly anxiety, depression, interpersonal difficulties and impairment of sexual relationships are frequent aftermaths of breast surgery.

Hysterectomy, like breast resection, for many women represents loss of a valued organ. This operation is discussed further in Chapter 8.

Learned dysfunction

In this type of dysfunction the initial stressful situation may no longer be operative, but the behaviour continues in a learned manner. Learned causes may be single or multiple. A single unpleasant episode in a vulnerable person may result in a continued pattern of sexual dysfunction.

Family attitudes

More often multiple negative associations with sexuality are evident.

Family attitudes in the early years of childhood are especially influential. The child whose parent(s) are embarrassed by their own nudity and obviously uncomfortable about the child's naked body will teach the child similar attitudes. Comfort about close bodily contact is learned early in life. The child whose parent dislikes 'cuddles' may also feel uncomfortable about bodily touch.

Discouragement of self-stimulation and genital exploration in childhood and adolescence may result in a lack of awareness of sexual needs and faulty ideas of anatomy. Acceptance of one's own sexuality is a necessary prerequisite for enjoyment of the sharing of that sexuality with another person.

The child may also become aware of parental conflicts over sex and the implications of separate beds or bedrooms. Loss of a parent in childhood may lead to later distrust of intimate relationships. The woman whose father 'ran off with another woman' when she was aged 2 and whose mother complains that 'men can never be trusted' may find it necessary to 'hold back' in her emotional and sexual relationships with her husband.

If mother is accused of having 'loose morals' her daughter may resolve to make sure she stays in control of her sexuality. Such 'control' may prevent adequate arousal or orgasm. Other traumatic episodes, such as exposure, assault and rape, may also have occurred.

Preparation for the menarche often reveals parental attitudes. The girl whose parent has explained to her what will occur in a positive manner will often respond to her first period with feelings such as 'Now I feel grown up' or 'I'm becoming a woman'. Where there has been no preparation the girl may feel she is 'bleeding to death'. She will often turn for advice to a neighbour or relative as she perceives she cannot discuss sexuality with her mother. Some girls receive no education about menstruation from anyone. At menarche they have merely been handed a sanitary pad and belt. School-friends are often equally uninformed.

'Wet dreams' may similarly result in much guilt and distress for the young man who is not informed of their nature and that they are a normal occurrence.

Another learning that may occur is that it is useful to ejaculate quickly in order to avoid 'getting caught'. For this reason a male may masturbate rapidly. Later, when intercourse occurs in 'forbidden' situations, such as on the parents' lounge or in the back seat of a car, it may also be necessary to ejaculate as fast as possible. This male may subsequently have difficulty with ejaculatory control.

Unwanted pregnancy, abortion and other gynecological problems may add to other unpleasant associations to result in a learned pattern of sexual dysfunction.

Religious orthodoxy

Some researchers have stated that religious orthodoxy is responsible for conditioning sexual dysfunction. They included orthodox religions such as certain Jewish sects and Roman Catholicism as imposing many prohibitions on sexual functioning. The result is an environment in which all sexuality must be inhibited until after marriage and even then some restrictions remain. Not surprisingly, some people fail to develop a sexuality which has been so inhibited for many years.

Intrapsychic conflict

Sexual dysfunction may be a manifestation of underlying psychological conflicts, often of major intensity. Sexual conflicts are often unconscious. Freud drew attention to the importance of sexual conflict in human behaviour. He was so impressed by the frequency of these sexual conflicts that he claimed they formed the basis of most psychopathology. This viewpoint perhaps reflected the extremely sexually repressive influences of the society in which he lived.

Conflict between the wish to enjoy sex and the unconscious fear of doing so has many sources. Causes of sexual conflict include religious and cultural influences which tend to equate sex with sin, restrictive childrearing and failure of adequate psychosexual childhood development. Conflict is manifest as considerable anxiety, severe sexual dysfunction, disturbed relationships with parents and other disturbances in the social adjustment of the individual.

SEXUAL ASSESSMENT

Assessment of sexual complaints is neither difficult nor time consuming. The aims of history-taking are to delineate and describe the presenting problem and to identify the major etiological factors involved and their relative contributions. The practitioner is then able to plan a management approach. This may involve further investigations, treatment of organic disorders, sexual or marital counselling by the practitioner or referral to specialist clinics.

Sexual Problems

Doctors are often uncertain as to how much detail of sexual behaviour they legitimately should seek when assessing sexual functioning. Clinical experience indicates that it is necessary to obtain details of all aspects of the patient's thoughts, associated feelings and actual behaviour with regard to sex. Questions asked frankly and without embarrassment by the doctor will be answered in a similar manner by the patient. It is necessary at times for the doctor to be prepared to use and be familiar with the different vernaculars which may be used by patients from different social, cultural and occupational backgrounds to describe their anatomy and sexual behaviour. The doctor's awareness of his or her own attitudes and feelings about sexuality and the patient's sexual concerns will determine the ease and ability with which the clinical interview is handled.

Another concern is whether to interview couples together or carry out individual assessments. It is well accepted that there is no such thing as an 'uninvolved' partner in any problem of sexual interaction and it is therefore important to include the partner in the assessment. Individual interviews provide the opportunity for disclosure of information that may not be offered if the partner were present. Assessment of the couple together provides vital information about the nature and dynamics of the relationship, which may complement or differ significantly from their individual descriptions. It matters little whether individual or joint assessment is carried out initially, so the practitioner may be opportunistic and see whoever has presented.

Sexual history

The following questions may facilitate history-taking. Their details and the order of questioning may be amended according to the patient.

Presenting problem

'Describe the problems you are having.'

'Has it always been like this? If not, for how long have you had this problem?'

It is important to detail the exact nature and duration of the sexual concern or dysfunction.

Details should be sought of the patient's level of sexual interest, ability to become aroused and maintain this, enjoyment of sex, orgasmic ability and frequency of coitus and whether there have been changes in these.

'Does your partner have any difficulties with...?' Record the patient's assessment of the partner's sexual functioning.

Childhood and development

'Where were you born and brought up?'
    'What religion were you raised as?'
    'How many were there in your family?'
    'How would you describe your childhood?'
    'Were your parents happy in their relationship?'
    'Describe your relationship with them.'

Relationships with parents and the parents' own relationship is particularly important in determining a patient's ability to develop trust and intimacy in adult relationships.

'Were you given any sex education?'
'Did you have any sexual experiences as a child or growing up?'
'Were you given any preparation for the first period?'
'How old were you at puberty, self-stimulation, wet dreams, first dating, first sexual experience?'
'Did you have any homosexual experiences or fantasies?'
'Did you have any unpleasant sexual experiences prior to your present relationship?'

These questions provide the patient with an opportunity to detail any negative experiences which may have occurred during development, especially those of assault and rape.

Current relationship

'Are there any other problems in your relationship besides the sexual one?'
    'How do you feel towards your partner?'

The presence or absence of warm, loving, positive feelings and any disharmony should be particularly sought. The pattern of communication and interaction of the couples is best assessed at joint interview.

Acceptance of own sexuality

'Have you looked at your sexual parts, explored your vagina, self-timulated, reached orgasm by self-stimulation?'
    'Are you ever aware of sexual thoughts or fantasies when there is no-one around?'

These questions help to determine how the problem may reflect the failure of the individual to become comfortable with and knowledgeable of his or her own sexual identity.

Sexual Problems

Medical history

'Have you had any serious illnesses or operations?'

Alcohol and drugs

'How much alcohol do you drink?'
   Determine the amounts of alcohol (and drugs) consumed both now and at the onset of the disorder.

Contraception

'What method of contraception are you using?'
   The utilization and acceptance of contraception should be determined.

Moods

'How would you describe your usual mood — do you usually feel sad, fearful, tense, confused or bright?'
   The clinician should assess mental status during the interview.

Obstetric history

Women should be asked: 'How many pregnancies have you had?'
   'Were there any problems with the labours/births?'
   Response to and outcome of all pregnancies and lactation are relevant. Many patients relate the onset of sexual dysfunction to a pregnancy.
   'Have you ever had any illness or operation affecting your breasts or genital organs?'

Insight

'What do *you* think is causing the problem? Do you feel there is anything wrong with any part of your body?'
   Fears of physical abnormality may be expressed, such as the vagina being too small to allow intercourse or that the penis is too small to fully satisfy the female.

Examination

General and genital examinations are needed to indicate whether or not there is any organic pathology contributing to the disorder. Gentle, sensitive examination often rapidly increases rapport. Further information is often forthcoming whilst the patient is still on the examination couch. The sentiment is that the doctor, having looked, now knows all anyway. There are therapeutic aspects of the examination, especially the reassurance of physical normality.

Examination in the presence of the partner is often beneficial when ignorance and anxiety are shared. Diagrams, mirrors and pelvic models may be used to explain normal and abnormal physical findings. Whilst examination is desirable, it is not always possible to proceed if the patient manifests extreme anxiety. An example is the woman who has severe vaginismus, where it may be preferable to delay any vaginal examination until the patient has been taught how to relax the vaginal muscles.

Investigations

Hormonal

Serum testosterone and prolactin assays are ordered for all males presenting with dysfunctions other than premature ejaculation. Follicle-stimulating hormone and serum estradiol levels are often useful in determining hormonal contributions to female sexual dysfunction associated with the menopause.

Local

Vaginal smear and culture may be necessary to exclude vaginal infection as a cause of dyspareunia.

Laboratory

Nocturnal penile tumescence recordings are useful in determining the importance of organic factors in erectile failure.

MANAGEMENT

After assessing the individual or couple by means of the guidelines outlined, further management will be determined by the following considerations.

Sexual Problems

Sexual dysfunction or abnormal expectations?

When the real difficulty is that of unrealistic expectations, the therapist may be able to allay concerns. By encouraging discussion of the patient's fears and misunderstandings, re-education as to the nature of sexuality is possible. It may sometimes be helpful to reinforce this approach with a book, or film viewing.

Is the sexual dysfunction symptomatic of another problem?

When a current cause of sexual dysfunction is present, therapy initially should be directed to the cause rather than the specific sexual concern. For example, when interpersonal difficulties are evident and both partners have made the commitment to improve the relationship, therapy is directed at improving patterns of communication and at helping them to

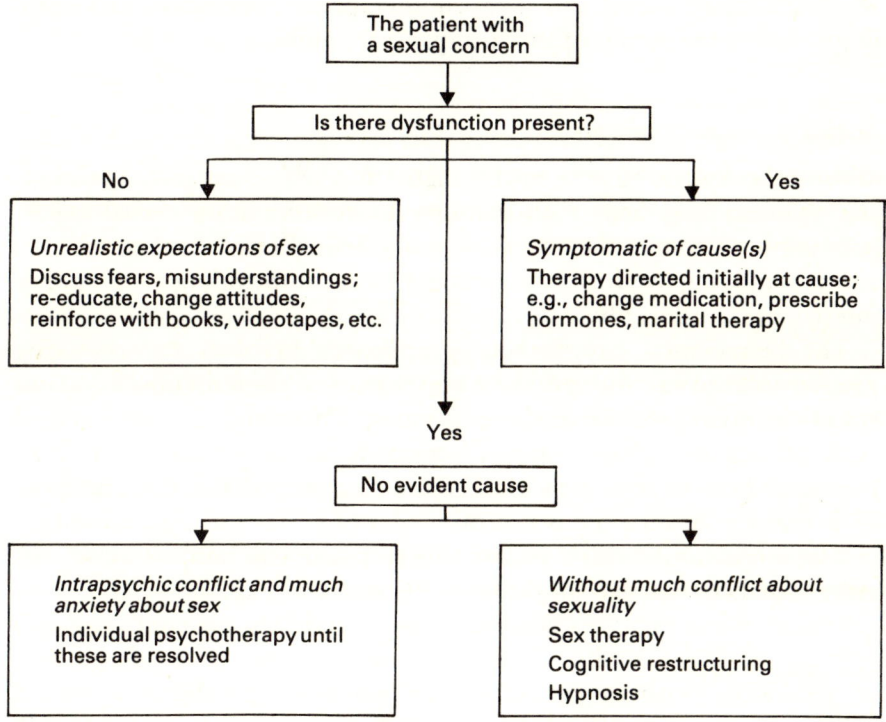

Figure 2   Management of sexual dysfunction

become aware of each other's needs. Therapy seeks to eliminate organic causes where possible, to increase utilization of restricted sexual capabilities, and to advocate the acceptance of those disabilities which cannot be altered. If other psychiatric disorders are present, therapy is focused on the underlying psychiatric illness. Pre-operative counselling of the patient and partner may help to prevent or lessen dsyfunction related to surgery.

Is there acceptance of one's own sexuality?

If the problem is a relatively minor one, it may be amenable to explanation and encouragement to explore and accept the genital area of the body. In others, there may be almost complete denial of the genital area of the body. Individual therapy is aimed at increasing the acceptance of total sexuality. Where the problem appears to be a learned pattern of behaviour, behavioural therapy techniques, such as systematic desensitization, are useful. Other psychotherapeutic approaches are helpful in producing resolution of any intrapsychic conflicts.

Sexual interaction problems

When other causes have been eliminated and self-acceptance is present, the problem may reflect an inability to communicate sexual needs. 'Conjoint' or couple therapy is essential here. Behavioural techniques aim at removing 'performance' anxiety by recommending avoidance of intercourse temporarily.

The behavioural psychotherapy approach involves tailor-making programmes to suit the specific requirements of the individuals and not simply applying standardized techniques. The couple are encouraged with the help of a programme of 'sensate focus' or pleasuring exercises to relearn how to arouse each other and to communicate their needs to their partner. Sensate focus is reminiscent of systematic desensitization in that it is assumed that a pleasurable response will become associated with sexual cues in place of the formerly occurring anxiety.

Sensate focus exercises heighten arousal and help the couple to start communicating sexually. These exercises consist of a programme of 'pleasuring', usually performed for half an hour a day in a relaxed setting. The couple are instructed not to have intercourse, in an attempt to remove performance fears and to enable them to relax and enjoy sensuality.

Pleasuring exercises are initially restricted to the non-genital area of the body. It may be suggested to the couple that a pleasant way to begin is to disrobe in a warm room and to give each other a soothing body massage with baby oil or powder. Talking about likes, dislikes and feelings is encouraged. The exercises may progress to the genital area and to individual preferences for reaching orgasm without penetration. This lessens anxiety over intercourse performance and may heighten the pleasure many couples achieve with sexual play. It is very important for the therapist to explore the couple's reaction to the instructions. The couple's reactions may be positive — they may experience sensations as sensuous and extremely pleasant and become optimistic about sexual relationships. At times there may be a lack of response or an adverse reaction. These reactions sometimes reflect marital disharmony or intrapsychic conflicts about sexuality.

Kaplan (1976) has further developed sex therapy by combining psychotherapeutic and behavioural techniques.

It is not possible to give a full account of the management of the many different types of sexual dysfunction in this short text. The reader is referred to one of the many volumes devoted to sexual therapy (see 'References and further reading).

CONCLUSIONS

Sexual assessment is neither difficult nor very time-consuming. Detailed questioning is needed so that the clinician can determine whether a disorder exists or whether the patient's concern reflects unrealistic expectations of sex, and then plan appropriate therapy. When there is an evident cause, therapy should be first directed towards this. Psychotherapeutic strategies (described in Chapter 2) are helpful in resolving conflicts about sexuality and restructuring attitudes to sexuality. Sex therapy techniques are based on behavioural strategies and help to reduce dysfunctional behaviour. The modern therapist employs a number of different treatment modalities, including understanding, communication, behavioural alteration, cognitive therapy, hypnotherapy, and, where appropriate, physical treatments and aids.

REFERENCES AND FURTHER READING

Davidsen, J, Kwan, M. and Greenleaf, W. J. (1982). Hormone replacement and sexuality in men. In Bancroft, J. *Clinics in Endocrinology and*

Metabolism, pp 599–624. W. B. Saunders & Co., London

Kaplan, H. S. (1974). *The New Sex Therapy*, Vol. I. Brunner/Mazel, New York

Kaplan, H. S. (1979). *Disorders of Sexual Desire: The New Sex Therapy*, Vol. II. Brunner/Mazel, New York

Kaplan, H. S. (1983). *The Evaluation of Sexual Disorders. Psychological and Medical Aspects.* Brunner/Mazel, New York

Masters, W. H. and Johnson, V. E. (1966). *The Human Sexual Response.* Little Brown & Co., Boston

Masters, W. H. and Johnson, V. E. (1970). *Human Sexual Inadequacy.* Little Brown & Co., Boston

Chapter 4

Contraception

INTRODUCTION

Throughout history all societies have shown some desire to control population growth. The limited methods available for the prevention of uterine conception (contraception) were supplemented in many communities by abortion and infanticide. One of the oldest known methods of birth control was coitus interruptus, withdrawal of the penis from the vagina before ejaculation. Genesis, 38:8-9, described how Onan 'spilled the semen on the ground, lest he should give offspring to his brother'. The Petrie papyrus of 1850 BC suggested as a contraceptive the use of a vaginal plug of crocodile dung and honey prior to coitus. Sea-sponges inserted as cervical barriers were also used in ancient Egypt. Cleopatra is said to have used a sea-sponge moistened with vinegar to prevent pregnancy.

Methods of contraception first used by the Greek and Roman civilizations included absorbent materials, root and herb potions, pessaries, and coitus interruptus. Surgical methods of contraception, such as sub-urethral incision, were used by primitive stone-age communities, such as the Australian aboriginal tribes. Oral medications said to affect fertility were prescribed in the 6th century Sanskrit books of instruction on love (the *Kama Sutra*) (Stopes, 1928).

Little is known of early contraceptive practices in Europe. By the middle of the 16th century penile sheaths made of fine linen had been introduced into Italy, apparently to reduce the risk of venereal disease. Sheaths were modified and refined. The 'condom', made of the dried gut of a sheep, was openly advertised and sold in 18th century London. Rubber condoms, cervical caps and cervico-uterine pessaries were introduced in the latter half of the 19th century (Stopes, 1928).

The 20th century has seen the development of chemical, mechanical and surgical methods of contraception, capable of providing a contraceptive effectiveness previously unavailable to mankind. In the last three decades there has been an unprecedented rise in the utilization of birth control techniques in both developed and Third World countries. In the United Kingdom over 95% of couples married in the 1970s used contraception at some stage in their marriages. The type of contraceptive utilized has also changed greatly during this time frame, increasing popularity of the more effective techniques of contraception. Thus, the pill and the intrauterine device (IUD) grew in usage, while the condom, coitus interruptus and the diaphragm were less popular. The publication of studies indicating adverse effects of the oral contraceptive pill on the cardiovascular system in 1977 (Vessey et al., 1977) led to increased concern over the effects of prolonged utilization of this method. Effects on the medical community include a revival of interest in other methods, refinements of these by new technology and pressure to develop new techniques.

There has also been increased recognition of the importance of motivational factors versus technical efficacy *per se* in determining fertility-regulating behaviour. In trying to understand the patient's individual needs in this regard it is important to examine the factors influencing contraceptive behaviours. This chapter will focus on the psycho-social aspects of contraception of most relevance to women.

REASONS FOR CONTRACEPTION

There are essentially two major arguments for using contraception, population pressure and personal reasons. The English economist and sociologist Thomas Robert Malthus (1766–1834) first sounded the alarm that if population growth continued unchecked by war, famine and disease, poverty and hunger were unavoidable. Though he did not suggest any means to limit population growth other than 'moral restraint', his warning spurred the beginnings of the birth-control movement in England. World-wide population growth has continued at an alarming rate. While it took until 1830 for the population of the world to reach one billion, this figure was doubled in the next century. It is predicted that if the world-wide population growth rate of 2% per year continues, the world population will double in thirty-five years. The primary reason for the staggering increase in population is a decrease in the death-rate, reflecting the advancement of medical technology.

Added to the problem of inadequate food production (with an estimated ten to twenty million people already dying of nutritional deficiencies annually) is that of consumption and pollution. These are related to affluence as well as population density.

The availability of modern efficient contraceptive technology has been effective in reducing population growth in the more affluent nations but has had little effect on the birth-rate of many of the developing nations of the Third World. This perhaps indicates the importance of considering personal incentives or contraceptive motivation.

Personal incentives include the prevention of illness, deformity and unwanted children. When serious genetic defects are present or there has been exposure to teratogenic substances, medical opinion tends to favour contraception, abortion or even sterilization. However, the overwhelming majority of peole in our Western society who utilize contraception do so to prevent unwanted pregnancy. The personal reasons involved may be to avoid a pregnancy out of wedlock or to postpone pregnancy for socio-economic, psychological quality of life and physical health reasons. The lack of success of birth-control programmes in some countries reflects little personal motivation for the individuals concerned. This especially applies to cultures where birth of many children is regarded as necessary to ensure the economic viability of the family unit.

It is obvious that socio-cultural, religious, psychological and sexual factors interrelate to influence contraceptive motivation, which in turn affects contraceptive acceptability.

FACTORS INFLUENCING CONTRACEPTIVE ACCEPTABILITY

Acceptability may be defined as that quality which makes an object, person, event or idea attractive, satisfactory, pleasing or welcome. Contraceptive effectiveness and acceptability are necessarily interwoven. For the first time in history we have available many contraceptive methods which technically are highly effective in preventing pregnancy. Use effectiveness is dependent on the couple involved having accepted and correctly used their contraceptive method. For example, the combined oral contraceptive pill is known to be almost 100% effective in preventing pregnancy if taken as directed. Unfortunately, prospective studies have demonstrated a high discontinuation rate in women prescribed the pill. While technical effectiveness of the pill is high, acceptability is not.

A universally acceptable method of birth control ideal for every age and life-phase is not available and is probably unachievable. Different techniques will be needed at different stages. Varying contraceptive situations include those of the teenager or young single adult who may be sexually active intermittently but wishes to avoid pregnancy; the young married couple who wish to space out pregnancies; the woman or couple who wish to curtail childbearing; and the woman in mid-life with altered life circumstances following separation or divorce who must reconsider her reproductive potential.

Effective contraception counselling requires consideration of all factors influencing choice of, motivation to use and ultimate acceptability of a contraceptive method. These factors include socio-cultural, intrapersonal and sexual aspects and knowledge of the side-effects (physical and behavioural) of the differing contraceptive methods.

Socio-cultural aspects

Government attitudes

The Government of a country may have a major authoritarian influence on contraceptive practice. Government policy may be influenced by religious pressure. The other important factor influencing Government policy is the economic problem of overpopulation. This has forced the Governments of India and China, for example, to provide cheap national programmes for birth control. In more affluent countries where population explosion is unlikely, the Government may influence contraceptive acceptability in a number of ways. These include support for community education aimed at improving contraceptive knowledge and the provision of free family-planning services for the lower socio-economic group. Government boards responsible for the licensing of pharmaceuticals influence the type of methods ultimately available to the public. Certain types of contraceptive methods may be subsidized to a greater or lesser extent under National Health schemes. This may result in financial barriers to long-term acceptability of a method not favoured by subsidy.

Cultural factors

Consideration of cultural factors may have spectacular benefits with respect to contraceptive acceptability improvement. A contraceptive clinic in Iran, a male-dominated society, achieved the excellent continuation rate of 93% for the oral contraceptive pill by making the male partner responsible for the woman's regular pill-taking (Siassi, 1972). In cultures such as this, where males hold dominant roles (for example, Italy), it may be more acceptable for the male to take responsibility for contraception. Male-oriented methods, such as the condom or coitus interruptus, may be preferred in these cultures. Some cultures have negative attitudes to vaginal insertion of the woman's own fingers. Methods requiring regular intravaginal insertion such as the diaphragm are likely to be less well favoured in these societies.

Social class

Social class differences may also influence contraceptive acceptability. The lower socio-economic groups may be more likely to take chances with contraception as life may seem unpredictable and a game of chance anyway. Childbearing may be one of the few sources of self-esteem available to the poor. Class barriers may also operate at contraceptive assessment, as most physicians have come from middle or upper socio-economic backgrounds. There may be difficulty in communication between patient and doctor, or because of different attitudinal systems the doctor may appear insensitive to the needs of the patient. Education has in itself been found to be conducive to the practice of contraception. An Australian study found that contraceptive practice increased with the number of years of education (Caldwell *et al.*, 1973).

Media

There can be little doubt that the media have a profound influence on contraceptive acceptability. Responsible reporting by the media can be of great benefit in improving the contraceptive and general health knowledge of the community. Perhaps the medical profession has a role to play in ensuring that suitable standards of medical reporting are achieved in the lay press.

Religious

Roman Catholic opposition to birth control is said to have evolved because of the threat of depopulation (Davis, 1971). The use of contraception and abortion by the Roman nobility, combined with high infant and adult mortality, resulted in a decline in the population of the upper class. The Catholic church and Roman state were further threatened by the introduction of a new religion, 'Manicheanism', which advocated celibacy and opposed procreation. After his conversion to Christianity, St Augustine turned against his former Manichean colleagues, making procreation the sole object and justification of intercourse. All forms of contraception, including coitus interruptus and the rhythm method, were considered sinful. This century has seen a softening of traditional Catholic attitudes to contraception, with the acceptance of the rhythm method and its refinements. Pope Paul's encyclical *Humanae Vitae* recognized the seriousness of unrestrained population growth, although simultaneously opposing, on Catholic moral principle, methods medically known to be the most effective for dealing with the problem (Callahan, 1968). The following translation of *Humanae Vitae* states the Catholic church's attitudes to contraception:

'. . . God has wisely disposed natural laws and rhythms of fecundity which, of themselves, cause a separation in the succession of births. Nonetheless, the church, calling men back to the norms of natural law . . . teaches that each and every marriage must remain open to the transmission of life.

The teaching . . . is founded on the inseparable connection, willed by God and unable to be broken by man on his own initiative, between the two meanings of the conjugal act, the initiative meaning and the procreative meaning.

The church is coherent with herself when she considers recourse to the infecund periods to be licit, while at the same time condemning, as always illicit, the use of means directly contrary to fecundation . . . In reality, there are essential differences between the two cases. In the former the married couple make legitimate use of natural disposition; in the latter, they impede the development of natural processes.' (*Humanae Vitae*, 1966. Paul VI in *The Catholic Case for Contraception*, edited by D. Callahan. Macmillan, London.)

Interestingly, a rising proportion of Catholics are employing birth control in many countries. In the USA the proportion of Catholic women using contraceptive methods other than rhythm increased from 30% in 1955 to 60% in 1970.

Other Christian churches: The Anglican Lambeth conference resolution in 1930 reversed the 1920 resolution which had condemned contraceptive practice. Most Christian churches now have favourable attitudes towards contraception.

Judaism: The Old Testament injunction 'be fruitful and multiply' (Genesis 1:28) is variously interpreted. One orthodox view is that a woman should have a minimum of one male and one female child. The *Talmud* advised the use of a mokh or woollen tampon to prevent pregnancy in minors or nursing mothers. Contraceptive practice is accepted by even the most orthodox if prescribed for 'medical reasons'. Most liberal sects accept contraception as an established part of modern living.

Muslim: The *Koran* attached high prestige to parents of large families but contained no specific prohibition of contraceptive practices.

Hinduism and Buddhism: There are no doctrinal obstacles to curbs on parenthood.

The attitudes of various religious faiths to contraceptive practice provide only a stereotype to the physician. Experience in contraceptive counselling suggests that the issue related to contraceptive acceptability is not the religious denomination *per se* but whether an individual will experience major conflicts with religious beliefs over the use of a particular contraceptive method. If conflicts and resultant anxiety are likely, it may be preferable to advise a method not in direct conflict with religious doctrine.

Intrapersonal

The intrapersonal approach to understanding sexual-reproductive behaviour focuses upon the interaction between psychosexual development as manifested in personality and the socio-cultural context. Brody and Newman (1983) describe how emotionally charged behaviours such as those involving sex and reproduction are strongly influenced by conscious and unconscious conflict involving variations of desire on one hand and internalized moral and judgmental standards on the other. The anxiety, guilt and shame generated by such conflict are dealt with by defence mechanisms which function mainly to keep unacceptable desires outside of consciousness or awareness. Whilst this reduces anxiety, guilt and shame to manageable levels, these emotions may break through in the form of behaviour which is often seen as impulsive or irrational. Such behaviours include those of impulsive intercourse, later regretted failure to contracept and sexual and reproductive risk-taking in general.

One example of such behaviour is represented by the increasing number of seemingly unplanned teenage pregnancies.

Teenagers in many Western countries are becoming sexually active at earlier ages. Although most have at some stage used contraception, over half those surveyed by Farrell (1978) admitted they did not always use birth control. The methods used showed a progression from the less reliable techniques at the beginning of sexual activity to more reliable methods by young adulthood. Thus the majority expose themselves to the risk of pregnancy at some stage.

Successful use of birth-control methods necessitates various decision-making and taking deliberate action to avoid pregnancy. Pregnancy can result from avoiding making a decision or postponing the necessary behaviour.

For effective use of contraception teenagers must first come to terms with the fact that they are going to be sexually active. They may have a romantic rather than realistic notion of love and sexual relationships. To plan to use contraception may be seen as ruining the romantic ideal of sex occurring spontaneously as the fulfilment of love. Traditional views of female pursuits may also play a role, with girls feeling that by planning to use contraception they may be declaring themselves as sexually available and to be disposed of.

It would seem sensible to encourage teenage boys, who operate under different social pressures, to take more responsibility for contraception. Neglect of teenage boys as a client group for contraceptive services is particularly short-sighted, as condom use by adolescents has important preventative health implications, in delaying the spread of sexually transmitted disease and helping to protect the cervix against changes which may lead to cervical cancer. In addition, adolescents have sexual intercourse infrequently. The daily protection offered by the pill may not be necessary. Use of the condom may help to avoid unnecessary consumption of hormonal preparations.

An example later in the life-cycle is that of the premenopausal woman's failure to contracept, resulting in an ambivalently received pregnancy which may represent an unconscious attempt to hold her youth, social desirability and husband (Brody and Newman, 1983).

In a somewhat different analysis of the 'contraceptive conflict', Luker (1975, 1977) applied cost-benefit analysis and behavioural decision-making theory. She argued that women are engaged in a constant re-assessment of the costs and benefits of contraception and pregnancy. The risk-taking set will also be influenced by the likelihood of pregnancy occurring and the subjective probability of reversing a pregnancy. Indirect influences include those of the social boundaries of motherhood, marriage pressures, consensual unions, family-building pressures, death of a significant other, pregnancy of a sibling and life transitions. The dynamic nature of the decision-making process was emphasized.

Sexual

It is impossible to separate contraception from sexuality, sexuality from the total personality and personality from the other psycho-social processes involved. Consideration of the psychosexual attitudes of the patient has often been inadequate.

For example, the sexually secure woman who accepts her own sexuality, is able to touch and look at her genitalia without uncomfortable feelings, and responds to and enjoys sexual relationships, will find many contraceptive methods acceptable. Other factors such as desired family size, religious attitudes, and physical suitability may help to determine her particular choice. As she enjoys sex she may have frequent coitus and be more likely to choose methods that are highly effective in preventing pregnancy.

The sexually insecure woman usually has inadequate knowledge and erroneous concepts of her own body, of sexual behaviour, and of contraception. There is often anxiety present during sexual interaction, which may manifest as vaginismus. It is important for the clinician to recognize this patient, as careful early management will help to prevent the continuation or the development of sexual problems. The sexually dysfunctional woman may be unable to accept her own sexual organs and is unlikely to choose a method requiring touch, such as the diaphragm. She may dislike any form of penetration, and may view insertive methods negatively. Her inadequate knowledge may result in false ideas, with fears of damage to the genital tract and cancer development common. She may be likely to discontinue oral contraception in the long term, as she does not see herself as benefiting from its use. In reality, she may be placed under increased demands for intercourse by her male partner now that the fear of pregnancy has been removed. As she does not enjoy sexual relationships, she may prefer her partner to take the responsibility for contraception. The use of the condom or coitus interruptus is encouraged by this woman, who may consider semen to be 'dirty and messy'.

Physical

Due attention must continue to be given to physical factors. A careful medical and menstrual history and general examination are necessary. These may help to suggest the range of contraceptives physically suited to the individual. For example, women with a past history of heavy, painful menses are not physically suited to IUD use. Recent findings of increased mortality of cardiovascular origin associated with use of the oral contraceptive pill suggest that women aged over 35 and who are smokers may be physically more at risk. A routine follow-up annual examination may also be desirable both to ensure that there are no physical side-effects of the therapy and to provide the opportunity for other prophylactic health measures, such as the detection of hypertension, breast tumours and cervical cancer.

While the importance of physical factors is emphasized, it should be remembered that failure to attend to the other factors influencing contraceptive acceptability may result in the high discontinuation rates observed.

The clinician

Clinicians' attitudes are important in influencing choice of, motivation to use and ultimate acceptability of contraceptive methods. All factors mentioned above also influence the physician to view some methods more favourably than others. The clinician's personal feelings and motivation influence perception of the patient's needs. Male middle-class medical professionals tend to have a high tolerance for deferred gratification and be predisposed towards forward planning and long-term goals. This may not be the usual social behaviour of working-class clients. Special problem areas include those of communication with the patient, religious views prejudicing attitudes to contraception, fixation by the clinician on a particular method, and maintaining an effective doctor-patient relationship. The social aspects of motivation to control fertility and contraceptive decision-making are often not considered. The doctor cannot divorce contraceptive behaviour from the rest of an individual's life.

Behavioural effects of contraceptive methods

A source of concern for both doctor and patient are the possible behavioural effects of the different contraceptive methods.

Use of barrier methods may have beneficial effects on some sexual relationships. The unsophisticated, sexually insecure woman prescribed the diaphragm may, by its regular use, increase her acceptance of her own vagina. Condoms eliminate the 'messy component' for some, and spermicidal agents provide extra lubrication.

Disadvantages include the decrease in spontaneity and delay. The condom is frequently claimed to interfere with the sensual pleasure of both partners. Many women object to the nuisance and aesthetic aspects involved in the repeated insertion, removal and cleaning of devices. Coitus interruptus may lessen the enjoyment of the sexual act for both male and female and may provoke anxiety or tension in the couple. It seems probable that some couples would find distressing the need to turn sexual behaviour on or off according to the fertile period rather than actual desire. Coitus-inhibiting methods require significant motivation, co-operation and intelligence.

Most studies of behavioural effects of contraceptive methods have focused on the pill. A large-scale demographic study (Westoff, 1974) found that women using the pill have higher coital frequency than women using other contraceptive methods. Whether this was cause or effect was not clear. Rice-Wray *et al.* (1963) reported that 54% of women pill-users interviewed reported an increase in coital frequency after commencing to take the pill.

Explanations for positive effects on sexual behaviour included the contraceptive efficiency of this method, which allowed separation of procreational sex from recreational sex, as well as the separation of the coital act from the contraceptive act. Many women reported increased relaxation and spontaneity in sexual relationships (Rice-Wray *et al.*, 1963). Another mechanism proposed to explain positive effects of the pill reflects the beneficial effects exerted on menstrual complaints.

Possible adverse behavioural effects of the oral contraceptive pill have received much attention in both the lay and medical press. When studies which investigated adverse effects were reviewed there was found to be a wide incidence of 'loss of libido' and mood changes reported (Dennerstein and Burrows, 1977). There were a number of common features in the studies which claimed a high incidence of 'decreased libido' or mood change. They were mostly retrospective (Kane *et al.*, 1967; Nilsson *et al.*, 1967). If they were prospective the duration of the study was short (for example, two months — Grounds *et al.*, 1970). Studies often involved a biased sample with over-representation of psychiatric patients. In the report by Kane and co-workers (1967), eleven of the fifty women studied were psychiatric in-patients. The sample size was sometimes so small that it invalidated the conclusions. A possible reason for the disparity in results may be that the placebo-controlled, larger, prospective studies attempted to measure and separate the pharmacological effects of the pill from psychological effects. Retrospective studies were unable to separate psychological and pharmacological properties.

In order to differentiate between psychological and pharmacological effects, the design of a study should ideally incorporate a number of features such as the presence of an adequate control group and random double-blind methodology. Other factors which may influence the results of such a study include: the bias of the patient population selected; the problem of defining and assessing mental and sexual adjustments; the natural frequency of signs and symptoms in the population being studied; the relationship between the investigator and the patient; the personality of the patient; and the motivation of the patient (Drill, 1974).

Psychological factors in some women reflect the symbolism of taking an 'anti-baby' pill, the something that stops sexual intercourse being followed by pregnancy and childbirth (Cullberg, 1972). Other expectations will confer additional meanings on the pill. These may reflect the woman's past experience with tablets generally, or the pill in particular, as well as the experience of her peer group, her sexual partners and the media. For a few women, removal of the fear of pregnancy may have an adverse effect on sexual response, where this fear had balanced sexual guilt. Taking the pill may daily stimulate conflicts for the woman with sexual anxiety (Raphael, 1975).

One measure of the incidence of some psychological propensities of the pill was provided in a study in which women were given a placebo and informed that they were receiving the oral contraceptive pill (Aznar-Ramos *et al.*, 1969). A 'decrease of libido' was found in 30% of the couples. As these women all had a relatively recent spontaneous abortion and desired pregnancy, this study may in part have reflected an unwanted 'anti-baby' effect of the pill.

Cullberg (1972) attempted to minimize psychological propensities by telling the woemn he studied that they would receive only weak female hormones to assess what effect they had on premenstrual symptoms. In this study there was no change in sexual behaviour when women receiving oral contraceptives were compared with a control group of women receiving placebo. Significantly more women became depressed while taking the pill than placebo.

The results of this study and other double-blind studies of the effects of the pill on behaviour were summarized by Dennerstein and Burrows (1986). It would appear that adverse changes were more likely to occur in the first few weeks of pill-taking. Contrary to clinical impressions that gestagen-dominated pills were more likely to result in depression (Grant and Mears, 1967), two double-blind studies suggest that estrogen-dominated pills were associated with more depression (Goldzieher et al., 1971; Cullberg, 1972). Cullberg observed that women who became depressed on estrogen-dominated pills tended to have a past history of premenstrual irritability. Another predisposing factor to the development of pill-induced depression was said to be a prior history of depression (Leeton, 1973). When women who had undergone bilateral oophorectomy were studied in a double-blind trial (Dennerstein et al., 1979, 1980), more women reported improved mood and increased sexual desire and pleasure when estrogen was taken, compared with placebo. This improvement was not evident when the progestogen (Norgestrel) was compared with placebo. These findings are in accord with those of animal experimentation.

Pharmacological mechanisms

Schildkraut (1965) suggested that depression may reflect a deficiency of catecholamines at adrenergic receptor sites in the brain. Conceivably, elevated levels of brain monoamine oxidase activity could result in a depletion of catecholamines. Some workers suggest that progesterone may induce monoamine oxidase activity. Grant and Mears (1967) reported increased endometrial monoamine axidase activity when a strongly progestogenic pill was used. Klaiber et al. (1971) found that plasma monoamine oxidase activity was higher when both an estrogen and a progestogen were given to amenorrheic women than when an estrogen alone was used. However, plasma or tissue monoamine oxidase activity may not necessarily reflect the activity of monoamine oxidase in the central nervous system. Furthermore, the double-blind studies reviewed failed to confirm the hypothesis that the more progestogenic pills would produce more depression.

Other workers have suggested that pill-induced depression may be caused by low levels of brain 5-hydroxytryptamine (Winston, 1973). Women taking the pill show a marked disturbance of tryptophan metabolism along the kynurenine-niacin pathway, with abnormally high urinary excretion of several metabolites, particularly xanthurenic acid

(Rose, 1966). Several enzymatic reactions in the pathway require pyridoxal phosphate, derived from vitamin B6, as a co-factor. A relative pyridoxine deficiency, as evidenced by impaired tryptophan metabolism, was present in about 80% of pill-users. It appears that the majority of pill-users are able to meet the increased demands for vitamin B6. A small group of women pill-users can nevertheless be identified who have low urinary 4-pyridoxic acid excretion, altered pyridoxal phosphate-dependent erythrocyte enzyme metabolism and low plasma pyridoxal phosphate levels. These features indicate a failure to compensate for the increased B6 requirements due to the pill — a 'true' vitamin B6 deficiency (Wynn et al., 1975). Adams et al. (1974) showed that correction of a true vitamin B6 deficiency by oral administration of pyridoxine hydrochloride improved the mood of depressed pill-users. No response to pyridoxine was found amongst depressed women with a relative deficiency of vitamin B6 in this double-blind study. The disturbance in tryptophan metabolism is claimed to reflect the estrogenic component of the pill (Winston, 1973). The small group of women who develop an absolute deficiency of vitamin B6 when taking the pill may represent a group who are biochemically susceptible to oral contraceptives.

Changes in sexual desire may occur secondarily to the depressed mood (Cullberg, 1972). Alternatively, alterations in sexual response may reflect direct effects of hormones on central monoamine transmission.

Another possible mechanism for hormonal contraceptives to affect sexual response is via a pheromonal pathway. Michael and Plant (1969) treated female rhesus monkeys with two types of oral contraceptives, a combined pill and a sequential formulation, for six to seven months each. There was a diminution in the sexual activity of the male monkeys. This was demonstrated by less mounting behaviour, a decrease in the number of ejaculations and a consequent increase in the thrusting necessary to achieve ejaculation. These effects were more marked with the preparation containing more progestogen.

CLINICAL IMPLICATIONS

Mention has been made of the possible influences of the doctor on choice of, motivation to use and ultimate acceptability of contraceptive methods. For effective contraceptive counselling it is important that the clinician involved has awareness of his own attitudes towards contraception and sexuality.

Principles of adequate contraceptive care include those of: ready accessability of services; availability of both male and female doctors and of lay contraceptive counsellors in an effort to reduce the problems of the social distance from the client; understanding the patient in his/her social context and life-phase; provision of information about the likely effects, beneficial and adverse, of all the available methods; allowing the patient/couple to make an informed decision. It may be necessary to help the patient to understand and/or identify goals and resolve conflicts related to sexuality and/or contraceptive use.

It is important to remember that a 'less effective' method used consistently is likely to prove more effective than a supposedly 'highly effective' method used inconsistently.

For those who are sexually active but not involved in a stable relationship the advantage of condoms in providing protection against sexually transmitted infections should be considered.

CONCLUSIONS

For the first time in history we have available many contraceptive methods which technically are highly effective in preventing pregnancy. Use effectiveness is dependent on the couple involved having accepted and correctly used their contraceptive method. Socio-cultural, religious, psychosexual and physical factors all influence contraceptive acceptability. Awareness of all these factors and of the possible effects of the different contraceptive methods will help the clinician in the role of contraceptive counsellor.

REFERENCES AND FURTHER READING

Adams, P. W. V., Seed, M. *et al.* (1974). Vitamin B6, depression and oral contraception. *Lancet*, **ii**, 516–17

Aznar-Ramos, R., Giner-Velazques, J., Lara-Ricalde, R. *et al.* (1969). Incidence of side effects with contraceptive placebo. *Am. J. Obstet. Gynecol.*, **105**, 1144–9

Brody, E. B. and Newman, L. F. (1983). Psychological aspects of personal fertility regulation. In Dennerstein, L. and Burrows, G. D. (eds) *Handbook of Psychosomatic Obstetrics and Gynaecology*, Vol. 15, pp 353–72. Elsevier Biomedical Press

Caldwell, J. C., Young, C., Ware, H. *et al.* (1973). Australia: knowledge, attitudes and practice of family planning in Melbourne, 1971.

Studies in Family Planning, **4**, 49-59

Callahan, D. (ed.) (1968). *The Catholic Case for Contraception.* McMillan, London

Cullberg, J. (1972). *Mood Changes and Menstrual Symptoms with Different Gestagen/Estragen Combinations.*

Davis, H. J. (1971). *Intrauterine Devices for Contraception.* Williams and Wilkins Co., Baltimore

Dennerstein, L. and Burrows, G. D. (1977). Sexuality and contraceptive acceptability. *Aust. Fam. Physician,* Special Issue, March, 19-22

Dennerstein, L., Burrows, G. D., Hyman, G. and Sharpe, K. (1979). Hormone therapy and affect. *Maturitas,* **1**, 247-59

Dennerstein, L., Burrows, G. D., Hyman, G. J. and Sharpe, K. (1980). Hormones and sexuality: effects of oestrogen and progestogen. *Obstet. Gynaecol.,* **56**, 316-22

Dennerstein, L. and Burrows, G. D. (1986). Effects of the oral contraceptive pill on mood and sexual behaviour. In Burrows, G., Norman, T. and Davies, B. (eds) *Drugs in Psychiatry.* Elsevier/North Holland Biomedical Press, Amsterdam

Drill, V. A. (1974). Some metabolic actions and possible toxic effects of hormonal contraceptives in animals and man. In Briggs, M. H. and Diczfalusy, E. (eds) *Pharmacological Models in Contraceptive Development,* Proceedings of WHO Symposium, Geneva

Farrell, C. (1968). *My Mother Said . . .* Routledge & Kegan Paul

Goldzieher, J. W., Moses, L. E., Averkin, E. *et al.* (1971). A placebo-controlled double blind cross-over investigation of the side effects attributed to oral contraceptives. *Fertil. Steril.,* **22**, 609-23

Grant, E. C. G. and Meares, E. (1967). Mental effects of oral contraceptives. *Lancet,* **ii**, 945-6

Grounds, E., Davies, B. and Mowbray, R. (1970). The contraceptive pill, side effects and personality: report of a controlled double blind trial. *Br. J. Psychiat.,* **116**, 169-72

Kane, F., Daly, R., Ewing, J. *et al.* (1967). Mood and behavioural changes with progestational agents. *Br. J. Psychiat.,* **113**, 265-8

Klaiber, E. L., Kobayashi, Y., Broverman, D. M. *et al.* (1971). Plasma monoamine oxidase activity in regularly menstruating women and in amenorrhoeic women receiving cyclic treatment with estrogens and a progestin. *J. Clin. Endocrinol. Metab.,* **33**, 630-8

Leeton, J. (1973). The relationship of oral contraception to depressive symptoms. *Aust. NZ J. Obstet. Gynaecol.,* **13**, 115-20

Luker, K. (1975). *Taking Changes: Abortion and the Decision not to*

Contracept. University of California Press

Luker, K. (1977). Contraceptive risk-taking and abortion. *Studies in Family Planning*, **8**, 190–6

Michael, R. P. and Plant, T. M. (1969). Contraceptive steroids and sexual activity. *Nature*, **222**, 579–81

Nilsson, A., Jacobsen, L. and Ingemanson, C. A. (1967). Side effects of an oral contraceptive with particular attention to mental symptoms and sexual adaptation. *Acta Obstet. Gynecol. Scand.*, **46**, 537–56

Raphael, B. (1975). Emotional factors in family planning. *Med. J. Aust.*, **2**, 943–5

Rice-Wray, E., Goldzieher, J. W. and Aranda-Rosell, A. (1963). Oral progestins in fertility control: a comparative study. *Fertil. Steril.*, **14**, 402–9

Rose, D. P. (1966). Excretion of xanthurenic acid in the urine of women taking progestogen-oestrogen preparations. *Nature*, **210**, 196–7

Schildkraut, J. J. (1965). The catecholamine hypothesis of affective disorders: a review of supporting evidence. *Am. J. Psychiat.*, **122**, 509–22

Siassi, I. (1972). The psychiatrist's role in family planning. *Am. J. Psychiat.*, **129**, 48–53

Stopes, M. C. (1928). *Contraception. Its Theory, History and Practice.* John Bale and Sons and Danielsson Ltd, London

Vessey, M. P., McPherson, K. and Johnson, B. (1977). Mortality among women participating in the Oxford/family planning association contraceptive study. *Lancet*, **ii**, 731–3

Westoff, C. F. (1974). Coital frequency and contraception. *Fam. Plan. Perspect.*, **6**, 136–41

Winston, F. (1973). Oral contraceptives, pyridoxine and depression. *Am. J. Psychiat.*, **130**, 1217–21

Wynn, V., Adams, P. W., Folkard, J. *et al.* (1975). Tryptophan, depression and steroidal contraception. *J. Steroid Biochem.*, **6**, 965–70

Chapter 5

Premenstrual Tension

INTRODUCTION

Mood and behavioural changes have been associated with the menstrual cycle since ancient times. A menstruating woman appears to have generally caused fear, evidenced in the taboos and regulations of many cultures. Ancient customs of the Yolngu aborigines called for menstrual isolation, dietary restrictions and a spiritual cleansing by being passed through the fumes of a smoky fire at the conclusion of menstruation. The Hebrews also isolated women during menstruation and for seven days thereafter and prescribed rituals for concluding the period of 'uncleanness.'

Menstruating women were credited with demonic powers in some cultures. The *Natural History* of Pliny (37–79 AD), Book VII, Chapter XV, asserts that such a woman sours wine, destroys the crops, dries the garden, makes fruit fall from the trees and kills bees.

The demonstration this century of the changing hormonal environment during the menstrual cycle has stimulated many studies attempting to correlate hormonal variations with behavioural and systemic changes.

AFFECTIVE VARIATIONS ACROSS THE MENSTRUAL CYCLE

The majority of women are probably aware of cyclical changes in mood and behaviour. The findings of twenty-four prospective studies of affective fluctuations during the menstrual cycle were summarized by Dennerstein and Burrows (1979). The majority of studies found that negative moods such as irritability, restlessness, anxiety, tension, migraine, sleep disturbance, impaired concentration, depression and increased neurotic conflicts were reported more frequently during the premenstrual and menstrual weeks. Although positive moods were not assessed as frequently as negative moods, the review suggested that increased feelings of well-being, elation, pleasantness and activation occurred during the follicular and mid-cycle phases.

PSYCHIATRIC DISORDERS AND MENSTRUATION

Until early this century menstruation and its abnormalities were considered to be important causes of psychoses. This etiological association has been eroded over recent years. Current classifications of psychiatric disorders, such as the American Psychiatric Association's D.S.M. – III, have no separate category for psychosis or abnormal behaviour recurring in close association with the menstrual cycle. The psychiatric literature contains scattered reports of patients with such cyclical psychoses.

The few detailed studies of patients with this disorder suggest that most sufferers are young unmarried women. In some cases the disorder became apparent during or soon after puberty. The psychotic episodes described commenced five to ten days premenstrually. Features included delusions, hallucinations, insomnia, hyperactivity, emotional lability, unusual behaviour and autonomic nervous symptoms such as flushing, anorexia or nausea. Following menstruation the symptoms diminished, with complete resolution during the interval period.

Increased rates of admission with acute psychiatric illness have been demonstrated in several studies. Dalton (1959) found marked increases of admission rates during the first four days of menstruation. The disturbing influence of menstruation appeared greatest amongst women aged less than 25 years. Abramowitz et al. (1982) found that 69% of depressed patients were admitted during the eight paramenstrual days ($p < 0.001$). 37% of schizophrenic patients were admitted during the paramenstruum ($p < 0.06$).

The possibility of a relationship between suicide (successful, attempted, or thoughts of) and the menstrual cycle has been explored by many workers. Most studies cited the menstrual phase as the most 'at risk' time. Several also cited the premenstrual phase and/or ovulation as times of high risk but less so than during menses. Others considered the late luteal phase as the time of greatest risk. One study found no relationship between suicide and the phases of the cycle but did observe that women were significantly more likely to attempt suicide in the second half of the cycle.

PREMENSTRUAL TENSION

The concept of a specific syndrome related to negative mood changes premenstrually was first introduced by Frank in 1931. He introduced the term 'premenstrual tension' to describe a specific and severe syndrome of unrest: irritability 'like jumping out of their skin', and 'a desire to find relief by foolish and ill-considered actions', occurring for the ten to seven days premenstrually, with complete relief after the onset of the menstrual flow.

Later authors have modified the syndrome in a number of ways. They have lengthened the number of cycle days affected. There has been disagreement about the phase of the cycle affected, with authors such as Dalton (1964) maintaining that symptoms could also occur at ovulation or during menses. The number and type of symptoms were also added to greatly. The recognition of associated physical and behavioural changes has led many authors to refer to a 'premenstrual syndrome' rather than to 'premenstrual tension'.

A major area of discussion between workers in this area revolves around whether symptoms disappear with the onset of menses or may be present throughout the cycle. Dalton (1980), in a letter to the *British Medical Journal*, distinguished between a premenstrual syndrome — 'the presence of symptoms always in the same phase of every menstrual cycle, together with a complete absence of symptoms for a bare minimum of seven consecutive days during the postmenstruum' — and menstrual distress — 'symptoms which increase during the premenstrual week but are present throughout the cycle come under the diagnosis of "menstrual distress"'.

Methodological problems

The failure to agree on a definition has led various investigators to utilize different criteria, creating much confusion in research into the relationship between the menstrual cycle and mood changes. This confusion has been further exacerbated by the inherent methodological difficulties in menstrual cycle research. An example is the diversity of assessment techniques used, often reflecting different and conflicting theories of behaviour. The validity of self-report as a tool to reflect the symptoms accompanying the menstrual cycle has been questioned by some workers. Few studies used a 'cover story' to minimize the subject's awareness of the investigator's objectives.

The greatest difficulty in interpretation relates to the differing and usually inadequate methods used to assign behaviour to menstrual cycle phases. Different methods have been used to organize data from cycles of disparate lengths. These techniques are based upon certain theoretical assumptions about the procession of hormonal events in cycles. One example is to use a standardized cycle of an arbitrary length, usually twenty-eight days, the assumption being that the pace of hormonal events is directly proportional to cycle length. Longer cycles are squeezed together, while shorter cycles are proportionately lengthened. Others have assumed that irregularities in cycle length occur before ovulation and that the time duration between ovulation and the onset of the next menstruation is a constant. The cycle phase is assigned by counting backwards from the onset of menses (reverse cycle day). 'If all women had the same length of menstrual cycle, with no inter- or intra-personal variance, and if hormonal events could be presumed to proceed in an invariant pattern during every cycle, the menstrual marker would be an adequate reference point for the association of behavioural observations and hormonal events. There is, however, no such regularity.' (Udry and Morris, 1977)

That the use of differing techniques may influence the results obtained is demonstrated in the study of Morris and Udry (1970). When pedometer readings were analyzed using reverse cycle day, no consistent change in physical activity was found. Significant changes in physical activity levels were evident on using the technique of standardized cycle day. The problem with these differing techniques which rely ultimately upon menstruation as the cycle marker is that little can be deduced about actual hormonal events within the cycle.

Udry and Morris (1977) suggested that fluctuations in steroid hormones and perhaps gonadotropins must be assessed during the menstrual cycle in order to correlate any changes in behaviour patterns with the variations in levels of ovarian and pituitary hormones. That hormonal changes might underlie certain affective changes was elegantly demonstrated by Somerville (1972), who studied six women who suffered a pattern of regularly recurring menstrual migraine. He demonstrated that falling levels of estradiol, rather than progesterone, in some way triggered off migraine in susceptible women. The migraine attacks were not affected by injections of progesterone but could be postponed by maintaining high plasma estradiol levels with injections of estradiol valerate.

Another important factor identified was that of adequate description of subjects so as to allow replication and comparison. Such description should, where possible, include age, race, country of birth, first language, occupation, marital status, parity, menstrual status and history, use of oral contraceptives and other medications, medical (including psychiatric) status and history and emotional stress prior to and during the study. These methodological problems are of importance when reviewing epidemiological and etiological studies.

Prevalence

Actual estimates of the incidence of the premenstrual tension syndrome have varied from 30–79%, depending on the definition of the syndrome, sampling procedures and method (Dalton, 1964). As most of these studies were based on retrospective reporting via questionnaire surveys, it is relevant to note that several authors have found discrepancies between retrospective reporting of menstrual cycle changes and actual findings from prospective data collected each day.

Etiology

Biological

A biological basis is suggested by the ubiquity of changes. An abnormality in the endocrine system has been sought to explain why some women are more severely affected than others.

Estrogen/Progesterone: An estrogen-progesterone imbalance and an excessive or deficient production of one or both hormones have been implicated as etiological factors in premenstrual tension, but the evidence has been conflicting. Frank (1931) reported symptomatic improvement in several cases following ovarian irradiation.

Low luteal phase levels of progesterone production, together with normal or high estrogen production, as measured by urinary or plasma analyses, were reported in premenstrual sufferers by some authors. In contrast, others found no such differences in plasma levels.

These conflicting results may be explained on the basis of insufficient sampling in each cycle (often only one or two measurements were made during the second half of the luteal phase), the use of small numbers of patients and controls and inadequate description of the subjects studied and of the diagnostic criteria used.

A study by Dennerstein *et al.* (1983a) has involved the collection throughout a complete menstrual cycle of 12-hour timed overnight samples of urine. Urinary total estrogens and pregnanediol were assayed. Patients consisted of thirty women referred with complaints of severe premenstrual tension, who were divided after an evaluation month into nineteen women with premenstrual syndrome and eleven women with menstrual distress. Results were compared with a control group of eighty-nine women without premenstrual complaints. This study found a 20% incidence of abnormal cycles (one anovulatory cycle, four cycles with short luteal phases and one cycle with low pregnanediol values during the luteal phase) in the patient groups, compared with an incidence of 4% in the control groups. Significantly lower pregnanediol values were found in the PMS patients during both the follicular and luteal phases of their cycles, compared with the matched and total controls. Asynchrony was observed between the first pregnanediol rise and the pre-ovulatory estrogen peak in the PMS patients, the pregnanediol rise occurring later than in the controls. These findings are at present unexplained. It remains uncertain whether the changes being observed are the result or the cause of PMS. If low progesterone is the cause of the symptoms of the premenstrual syndrome then progesterone therapy could be expected to relieve such symptoms. Dalton (1964) has long claimed the therapeutic efficacy of progesterone for such symptoms.

Whilst uncontrolled studies have reported favourable results, most double-blind studies failed to demonstrate any efficacy of progesterone over that of placebo. These studies have been criticized on the basis of the criteria utilized to select the sample and of the methods of assessing change in symptoms. A double-blind randomized cross-over trial of oral micronized progesterone (two months) and placebo (two months) was conducted to determine whether progesterone alleviated premenstrual complaints (Dennerstein *et al.*, 1985). Twenty-three women were interviewed premenstrually prior to therapy and each therapy month. They completed the Moos Menstrual Distress Questionnaire, Beck Depression Inventory, Spielberger State Anxiety Inventory, Mood Adjective Checklist and Daily Symptom Records. Analyses of data found an overall beneficial effect of being treated for all variables except restlessness, positive moods and interest in sex. Maximum improvement occurred in the first treatment month. Nevertheless, a significant beneficial effect of progesterone over placebo for mood and some physical symptoms was identifiable after both one and two treatment months.

There are many possible explanations for the positive findings in the present study when compared with those of other double-blind trials. In the present investigation the sample was studied prospectively before admission to the clinical trial. Although this reduced the sample size, there was objective evidence that the sample included in the clinical trial suffered from a discrete premenstrual syndrome. Great care was taken during the study to interview patients and have questionnaires completed each premenstruum, rather than relying on retrospective accounts which might have reduced the sensitivity of rating scales. Therapeutic effects can best be evaluated if the measuring instruments are valid, reliable and sensitive to change. For this reason a number of rating scales were utilized. Previous trials have administered progesterone by vaginal or rectal routes. It is possible that oral administration of progesterone might have produced more beneficial results than alternative routes. Further studies are needed to clarify whether this is so and to determine whether similar plasma levels of progesterone and its metabolites occur with each method of administration. Of interest would be the 5B reduced metabolite, pregnanolone, which appears to be responsible for the well-known hypnotic effect of progesterone.

Other evidence for the possible roles of estrogen and progesterone came from studies of the effects of the oral contraceptive pill. Women taking this pill complain of fewer premenstrual symptoms than do non pill-users.

Cullberg (1972) found no significant effect of the pill on premenstrual irritability or depression but did identify a small group of premenstrual tension patients made worse by highly estrogenic pills and better by strongly progestogenic ones. Morris and Udry (1972) found no difference in daily self-rated feelings of well-being when pill-users were compared with placebo-takers. Two other studies found that pill use eliminated cyclical changes in performance tests.

Prolactin: Halbreich et al. (1976) noted that prolactin caused water, sodium and potassium retention; was increased during the premenstrual phase of the cycle; was not changed by hysterectomy or the menopause and was thus applicable as an explanation for women who continued to experience cyclical changes after these events; was increased during the third trimester of pregnancy when toxemia was more common and was increased by stress. These workers found serum prolactin to be higher throughout the menstrual cycle in premenstrual sufferers than in controls. Other workers found that prolactin levels tended to be higher in premenstrual sufferers with low progesterone levels.

Three double-blind studies found bromocryptine to be significantly more effective than placebo in relieving some premenstrual symptoms.

It is not clear whether this reflected suppression of prolactin levels or other effects of bromocryptine, such as dopamine agonist actions.

Raised serum prolactin might reflect altered monoamine levels in the central nervous system. Monoamine oxidase activity has been shown to vary cyclically in both animals and man, being highest during the luteal phase. More recently, premenstrual symptoms have been attributed to luteal phase sensitivity and subsequent withdrawal from the neuropeptides beta-endorphin and alpha-melanocyte stimulating hormone.

Aldosterone: Excessive aldosterone action due to a lowered progesterone has been suggested to explain the accumulation of fluid premenstrually (Dalton, 1964). The affective changes may then be secondary to edema or perhaps reflect a substance fluctuating in parallel with aldosterone, such as angiotensin.

No consistent difference in aldosterone levels was found when women with premenstrual syndrome were compared with controls. Researchers have also failed to find a consistent relationship between fluid retention and premenstrual complaints. O'Brien *et al.* (1979) found that spironolactone reduced weight and relieved psychological symptoms in 80% of the symptomatic group studied. Further evaluations are needed to determine if this effect will persist over many months.

Pyridoxine: Pyridoxine in the form of pyridoxal-5-phosphate is a cofactor in a number of enzyme reactions in the body, including two pathways leading to dopamine and serotonin production. A deficiency of pyridoxine could then lead to decreased serotonin and depression and to decreased dopamine. Dopamine acts as a prolactin-inhibiting factor and increased prolactin would thus result, leading to effects on fluid balance and the breast. Although the use of pyridoxine in the treatment of premenstrual tension has shown impressive results on an informal basis, there was little evidence for pharmacological actions in better controlled studies. At present in the popular press there is great enthusiasm for such therapy. Scientific evidence is still needed. Unfortunately, virtually no work has so far been carried out on pyridoxal phosphate levels in blood. Such techniques are necessary to demonstrate whether or not premenstrual sufferers are deficient in pyridoxine.

Prostaglandins: Other substances fluctuating in parallel with the menstrual cycle might play a role in the etiology of affective changes. Few of these have been investigated to date. Prostaglandins are now known to affect many organs, including the brain, kidney, bowel and uterus. A double-blind cross-over study (Wood and Jakubowicz, 1980) found the anti-prostaglandin, mefenamic acid, to be significantly more effective than placebo in relieving premenstrual complaints. There were some methodological problems in this study in relation to adequate definition of the sample and the high co-existence of dysmenorrhea.

Psycho-social

Etiological theories range from the essentially biological to those that are basically psychological. Because the syndrome is complex, it is difficult to concentrate on one to the exclusion of the other. It is clear that in the majority of premenstrual syndrome sufferers there are psychological factors exacerbating the problems.

This section considers how such factors may operate and why some women cope with menstrual cycle changes while others do not.

Social-learning: Cyclical changes in affect may be socially learned. In a study of 255 women, Paulson (1961) found that 58% of the 'high premenstrual tension' group had mothers who suffered painful menstruation and premenstrual dysfunction, while only 27% of the 'low premenstrual tension' group had symptomatic mothers. The vital part played by cognitive factors in responding to bodily changes and feelings has been cited in previous chapters. The term 'attribution' is used to describe the process by which a person assigns blame or makes a causal inference about events. An attributional pattern, linking negative mood swings to the approach of menstruation, has been demonstrated. Further evidence of the influence of psycho-social factors on menstrual-related symptoms was provided by Ruble (1977). She found that women who were led to believe that menses were due in one to two days reported a higher degree of distressing symptoms than did those who believed they were intermenstrual. The two groups studied were in fact at identical phases of their menstrual cycles.

Paulson (1961) reported a tendency toward increasing negative attitudes toward self to be associated with increased premenstrual tension. The most highly distressed women have been found to be shy, self-doubting, eager to seek help from others and self-defeating. Cyclical variations might also be a factor in attitudes toward self. Higher self-esteem scores have been found associated with the ovulatory peak in estrogen during the menstrual cycle.

A woman's acceptance or rejection of her 'feminine role' has been investigated in several studies of the premenstrual syndrome. The results have been contradictory. Many researchers have maintained that women indicating greater distress premenstrually both resent and do not accept the traditional feminine role. Conversely, other investigators have found that more traditional and conservative women scoring high femininity scores have shown the greatest distress.

Personality: Some researchers have found that a tendency to develop the syndrome is related to personality type and a tendency to complain of other symptoms. The 'premenstrual syndrome woman' has been found to have personality characteristics of instability and suspicion, is guilt prone, apprehensive, unpretentious, tense, with much self-conflict. A greater part of the premenstrual research literature has shown a strong association between premenstrual tension and neuroticism.

Women with premenstrual complaints were more likely to be separated or divorced, without children, non pill-users, with sexual and emotional difficulties and dissatisfied with work.

This indicates that the 'premenstrual syndrome woman' generally shows an inability to cope successfully with environmental stress or the added stress from internal changes.

Whether such factors were the result or the cause of premenstrual complaints was not discernible. However, the psychological factors reviewed are likely to be important in providing effective total management of women presenting with premenstrual complaints.

IMPLICATIONS FOR THE CLINICIAN

Assessment

The first major problem facing the clinician is making a diagnosis. All patients presenting with premenstrual complaints need a full assessment. This requires interviews, examination and some quantification of symptomatology to be carried out in both the follicular and premenstrual phases of the cycle. Simple assessment methods may include a Daily Symptom Rating Scale (see Table 3) or the Moos Menstrual Distress Questionnaire.

In routine clinical management hormonal evaluation is seldom needed. Weekly determinations of ovarian steroids and gonadotropins may be helpful in the assessment of the woman with amenorrhea and

Table 3

A DAILY SYMPTOM RECORD CHART

Week beginning: _____

Name: _____

My last period started on: _____

Each night before retiring, please record your experience during the day of the feelings and sensations listed below. Write a number in the box opposite the item to indicate how intensely this symptom or feeling was experienced.

```
    1           2           3            4           5
    |           |           |            |           |
   Not         Very      A moderate    A fair     A great
  at all      little      amount        bit        deal
```

Date					
1. Restlessness					
2. Headache					
3. Breast discomfort					
4. Depression					
5. Active aggression					
6. Hot flushes					
7. Feelings of well-being					
8. Irritability					
9. Sexual thoughts or interest					
10. Swelling of abdomen, hands, legs					
Menstruation — number of pads or tampons used					

cyclical complaints, or for the perimenopausal woman. Prolactin estimations are necessary only if a pituitary lesion is suspected; for example, in a woman with galactorrhea.

Some patients appear improved by the process of assessment and state that no further therapy is required. Other women will be identified who, despite self reports to the contrary, do not appear to have a significant increase in symptomatology premenstrually. These patients should be treated for their primary psychiatric diagnoses. The remaining patients will consist of two groups: those with a discrete premenstrual syndrome and those with symptoms of some type throughout the cycle which may be exacerbated premenstrually. In the latter group psychological factors appear more important, whereas in the PMS group hormonal factors are more marked.

Treatment

A broad approach should be taken to planning therapy. Our research results indicate both psychological and hormonal factors might be important in premenstrual symptomatology. There are as yet no studies indicating whether the various therapy approaches might be differentially effective.

Information

After the assessment the results should be explained to the individual patient and a rationale for her symptoms offered. A general rationale would explain that psychological or thinking patterns, hormonal abnormalities and individual sensitivity to hormone-provoked symptoms are all important in the genesis and maintenance of symptoms. The role of each of these in the individual presentation can then be highlighted.

Intervention

There is little substantive evidence of the effectiveness of the widely used medications, pyridoxine and diuretics. Most patients attending our clinics had already received these medications and reported little improvement. There was initial resistance to psychological therapy approaches. Most patients seem to desire hormonal intervention. Hormonal intervention with oral micronized progesterone 100 mg in the morning and 200 mg at night from day 17 to 27 is recommended. In contrast, the 19-norsteroids often worsen premenstrual complaints.

Once an initial improvement in symptomatology has been achieved, women often become much more accessible to psychological treatment strategies. Supportive therapy and techniques aimed at increasing coping skills (and changing dysfunctional cognitions) are likely to be helpful. Behavioural techniques such as relaxation and assertiveness training might also be helpful.

The beneficial effects of combined therapies were demonstrated in a study by a co-worker (Morse and Dennerstein, 1986). Following the trial of oral progesterone some of the women continued hormonal medication and participated in a group treatment programme which utilized rational emotive therapy and relaxation training. A further improvement in symptomatology (mood, behaviour and pain), cognitive functioning and neuroticism was effected. Hormonal therapy was then withdrawn. Follow-up three months later showed that improvements in mood were maintained but not in symptoms of pain and water retention. This study demonstrated that the combination of cognitive behaviour therapy with hormonal intervention produced a more substantial reduction in PMS symptoms that did drug treatment alone.

REFERENCES

Abramowitz, E. S., Baker, A. H. and Fleischer, S. F. (1982). Onset of depressive psychiatric crises and the menstrual cycle. *Am. J. Psychiat.*, **139**, 475–8

Cullberg, J. (1972). Mood changes and menstrual symptoms with different gestogen/estrogen combinations. *Acta Psychiat. Scand.*, **(Suppl.)**, 236

Dalton, K. (1959). Menstruation and acute psychiatric illness. *Br. Med. J.*, **1**, 148–9

Dalton, K. (1964). *The Premenstrual Syndrome*. William Heinemann Medical Books Limited, London

Dalton, K. (1980). Letter to the Editor: Progesterone, fluid and electrolytes in premenstrual syndrome. *Br. Med. J.*, **2**, 61

Dennerstein, L. and Burrows, G. D. (1979). Affect and the menstrual cycle. *J. Affec. Dis.*, **1**, 77–92

Dennerstein, L., Spencer-Gardner, C., Brown, J. B., Smith, M. A. and Burrows, G. D. (1983a). Premenstrual tension — hormonal profiles. *J. Psychosomat. Obstet. Gynaecol.*, **3**, 37–51

Dennerstein, L., Judd, F. and Davies, B. (1983b). Psychosis and the menstrual cycle: A case report. *Med. J. Aust.*, May 28, 524–6

Dennerstein, L., Spencer-Gardner, C., Gotts, G., Brown, J. B., Smith, M. A. and Burrows, G. D. (1985). Progesterone and the premenstrual syndrome: a double-blind cross-over trial. *Br. Med. J.*, **290**, 1617–21

Frank, R. T. (1931). The hormonal causes of premenstrual tension. *Arch. Neurol. Psychiat.*, **26**, 1053–7

Halbreich, U., Assael, M., Ben-David, M. and Bornstein, R. (1976). Serum-prolactin in women with premenstrual syndrome. *Lancet*, **ii**, 654–6

Morris, N. M. and Udry, J. R. (1970). Variations in pedometer activity during the menstrual cycle. *Obstet. Gynecol.*, **35**, 199–201

Morris, N. M. and Udry, J. R. (1972). Contraceptive pills and day-by-day feelings of well-being. *Am. J. Obstet. Gynecol.*, **113**, 763–5

Morse, C. and Dennerstein, L. (1986). Cognitive perspectives of premenstrual tension. In Dennerstein, L. and Fraser, I. (eds) *Hormones and Behaviour*, pp 197–203. Excerpta Medica, Amsterdam

O'Brien, P. M. S., Craven, D., Selby, C. and Symonds, E. M. (1979). Treatment of premenstrual syndrome by spironolactone. *Br. J. Obstet. Gynaecol.*, **86**, 142–7

Paulson, M. J. (1961). Psychological concomitants of premenstrual tension. *Am. J. Obstet. Gynecol.*, **81**, 733–8

Ruble, D. N. (1977). Premenstrual symptoms: A reinterpretation. *Science*, **197**, 291–2

Somerville, B. W. (1972). The role of estradiol withdrawal in the etiology of menstrual migraine. *Neurology*, **27**, 355–65

Udry, J. R. and Morris, N. M. (1977). The distribution of events in the human menstrual cycle. *J. Reprod. Fertil.*, **51**, 419–25

Wood, C. and Jakubowicz, D. (1980). The treatment of premenstrual tension with mefenamic acid. *Br. J. Obstet. Gynaecol.*, **00**, 000–00

Chapter 6

Infertility

INTRODUCTION

In most cultures pregnancy and parenthood represent critical and desirable developmental phases. Involuntary infertility is understandably regarded as a cause of much distress and marital unhappiness. Some 15% of the population of childbearing age will be unable to achieve pregnancy and live birth. Medical science has made huge advances in the investigation and treatment of many of the disorders which can cause sterility. This progress in the field of reproductive medicine appears to have focused almost entirely on biology. Little attention has been given to psychological factors. Failure to appreciate psycho-social aspects has led to complaints and fears that new technologies are analogous to baby factories. *In-vitro* fertilization (IVF) is seen as another technological advance which results in doctors carrying out procedures on women's bodies, ignoring the human aspects of the problem.

For both gynecologist and the infertile couple the objective is to find a cause of the infertility and institute a treatment that will lead to the birth of a healthy child. Unlike other forms of medical care, which are usually directed at the cure of a disease, the management of infertility is aimed primarily at the attainment of a social achievement. In infertility, 'medical' disorder interferes with attainment of a basic need or life goal. Psychological factors are likely to be of especial importance in modulating or exacerbating the course of infertility and the couple's reaction to it. The unusually long period of treatment and the number of therapeutic interventions, combined with the central importance of fertility to personal identity, have implications for the doctor-patient relationship. The psychosomatic approach is of particular importance in infertility management. The gynecologist who understands the couple's feelings during their infertility will help to lessen their distress as well as his own frustrations.

This chapter examines some of the ways in which psychological and organic factors intertwine, with emphasis on the implications for the clinician.

THE MEANING OF INFERTILITY

The desire to reproduce, have and nurture children is a basic or instinctual need. Like our other needs, the wish for children is influenced by psychological and social factors. Intrapersonal factors include the individual's own experience of being parented. The person who has enjoyed love, trust and nurturing during development will look forward to sharing similar experiences with his own family. Those indivuals whose basic needs were not met during childhood may seek to make up for their deprivation by becoming parents themselves. A few will have been so damaged emotionally during childhood that they will consciously or unconsciously delay or reject parenthood. The desire to have a child is a dynamic one and thus will be influenced by the individual's environment. A harsh or adverse social environment might reduce the desire to parent in some, while others will view a child as a consolation. A major factor for many is the presence of a secure interpersonal relationship. 'Out of love grows love' is the adage. Yet some also seek to parent because there is no love (or relationship). Social and cultural factors also affect the desire to parent. Becoming a parent is highly valued by most societies. Modern Western society emphasizes role choice for individuals and there is less social stigma placed on the childless than in previous generations. The perceptual link between sex-role identity (as masculine or feminine), fertility and potency or sexuality remains. Consequently many women and men feel 'incomplete' if unable to parent.

The feelings of the couple and the gynecologist and their interaction will vary with the phase of infertility management. Let us consider the psycho-social aspects of the infertility life history of a couple.

Discovery of failure to become pregnant

Some women and men suspect or are aware that they will be infertile. Examples include those who have had genetic or congenital abnormalities diagnosed during childhood or adolescence. While the impact of infertility is no less intense, these individuals may structure their future lives and relationships with the knowledge of infertility. Others may be informed of the likelihood of later infertility following the diagnosis of disorders such as endometriosis or pelvic inflammatory disease. The majority discover infertility when conception fails to occur. With an increasing tendency of couples in Western society to marry later and postpone first childbirth for career and economic considerations, many couples do not discover their infertility until their third decade. The timing of the discovery of infertility has an additive effect on the personal meaning of childlessness. There is often a 'pressure-cooker' effect to demands for investigation and treatment when infertility is discovered in a woman in her mid or late thirties.

Infertility evokes many different feelings in the couple. These may vary in order and intensity. Many do not experience the full impact of the meaning of infertility until they have exhausted treatment avenues. Infertility may then be experienced as a crisis.

The first reaction of most people to the discovery of infertility is that of shock and surprise. Society tends to regard fertility as a given, to be controlled until children are desired. There is little preparation for the possibility of infertility. Denial is often the next reaction. This can be helpful in allowing the mind to adjust gradually to the impact of infertility, but it is dangerous when it becomes the major or permanent coping mechanism. Other common feelings experienced initially are those of frustration, humiliation and failure. These feelings are readily understandable in the perspective of the couple who have not achieved the pregnancy they believed would occur naturally once contraception was ceased.

The infertility investigation

Although in the majority of cases the investigation of an infertile couple includes very simple procedures (sperm analysis, post-coital test, basal body temperature (BBT), hysterosalpingography (HSG), laparoscopy), it must be kept in mind that the burden for the patients might be much heavier than the doctor imagines. This holds especially for female investigation. There is a great discrepancy between prescribing and undergoing a procedure. Many gynecologists do not realize what it means for a woman not only to undergo a pelvic examination, but also to keep BBT recordings month after month and have repeated post-coital tests performed — both of which can affect the social and sexual life of the couple. HSG, which usually is, as it should be, performed on an out-patient basis in the cold and technical atmosphere of a radiology department, combines humiliation, pain and fear, and laparoscopy usually means hospitalization and general anesthesia. Both procedures evoke ambivalent feelings of hope that some treatable cause will be found and fear that a serious untreatable abnormality will be exposed. These investigations have effects on the person, partner, and the relationship.

The majority of couples report deleterious effects on their sexual relationships. Both members of the couple are subjected to performance pressures. Aspects of sexual functioning which previously occurred spontaneously in response to loving and erotic feelings now occur in response to clinical demand. Complaints that sex has become cold, too purposeful and lacking in spontaneity are common. Some men and women lose interest or ability to become aroused under these circumstances.

Anger is a predictable response of the infertile couple to the frustration, helplessness, embarrassment and the surrendering of control of their bodies to the doctor. Excessive anger is sometimes a defence against intense pain and grief which the individual cannot yet acknowledge. The situation is made difficult for the couple as their feelings of anger are often directed at the gynecologist and yet they know rationally that the gynecologist is their only source of salvation. No wonder that the infertile patient often seems emotional, easily upset and demanding. Anger tends to dissipate with the opportunity to talk about it. Recognition and acceptance of the couple's feelings and the opportunity to discuss feelings, with a member of the infertility team or in a peer support group, can be of great benefit.

Infertility is often difficult for most people to discuss with others in their social network as it is both personal and inherently sexual. Many keep their infertility secret, even from members of their families. This may cut the couple off from sources of support at a time when such help is needed. In some cases infertile couples become so sensitive to issues of pregnancy or young children that they withdraw from social situations in case they are confronted by such contact. Increasing isolation may result.

Another reason for the secrecy which so often accompanies infertility is guilt. It is not unusual for an individual to search the past for a deed for which punishment in the form of infertility is now being extracted. Common guilt producers include premarital or extramarital sex, contraception, abortion, veneral disease, masturbation, and homosexual thought or acts.

Female infertility

When the infertility investigation reveals a female cause, a special situation arises. Despite emancipation processes in most Western societies, the majority of couples have a fairly traditional sex role distribution: the woman is supposed to become pregnant and to have, nurture and bring up children while the man works and provides the necessary income to maintain his family. When the probable cause of infertility lies in the female partner, her already damaged feeling of self-esteem will be reinforced by feelings of failure and guilt because she is unable to comply with the social expectancy and, moreover, the inability is her fault. The husband might say: 'I do not care so much; I have my work and the social contact it involves, but it is terrible for my wife because she is so alone.' And the wife might say: 'My husband was unlucky to marry me because I cannot give him what he deserves: a child.' Such statements reflect an unfortunate reality, which is further intensified by the general tendency to underestimate the value of housework, thus also giving the woman a strong feeling of being useless.

Gynecologists, who in terms of their speciality might be expected to *help* women, should be aware of these feelings and take a positive attitude toward the emancipation of women at the individual and public levels. The emancipated and working woman with a partner who shares and respects these views may have less difficulty in coping with and eventually working through their infertility — which of course does not mean that grief is less intense.

Male infertility

When the infertility investigation reveals a male cause, the resulting situation is in some ways similar — as far as the general and social consequences are concerned — but has very specific aspects at the individual level. Whereas female infertility generally does not affect the woman's sexuality, the opposite is much more likely in male infertility. In our culture, fertility, masculinity, and potency are closely related. The traditional linkage of sexuality and reproduction seems to be stronger amongst men than women. Whereas the infertile woman will tend to have feelings of failure and uselessness, infertile men tend to have feelings of not being a man and, even more so, of no longer being a sexual man. It is probably for this reason that there still is a taboo on male infertility, which has historically been kept masked in order to preserve 'masculine pride'. Female partners of infertile men sometimes say: 'I am so sorry for my husband; I would rather the fault was mine.' The reverse is very seldom heard. The male factor was long excluded from the infertility investigation, and fertility research focused mainly on the female.

Even now, there is still a general tendency among the public to look at the woman when a couple remains childless, although it is well known that the male factor plays a part (either totally or partially) in approximately 50% of the infertile couples. In this respect it is interesting to note how long it has taken the medical profession to overcome its aversion to artificial insemination with donor sperm (AID) compared with the ease and public openness with which *in vitro* fertilization and embryo transfer have been accepted. It is important to realize how peculiar the AID situation is: the 'treatment' of male infertility is in practice directed at the female partner, and the real cause of the infertility remains a secret hidden from the outer world.

Most of the couples in AID groups have reported a significant decline in sexual activity, and sexual pleasure had often disappeared. The women indicated that they no longer saw the purpose of intercourse, and the men said they could abstain for weeks. Some men said they had completely lost sexual interest after learning about their infertility, and one of them reasoned as follows: 'Since I cannot give proof of my manhood, I even have less sex than I want, as a punishment for myself.' On the other hand, men appeared to be relieved at discovering that other infertile men in the group had a distinctly masculine appearance, being tall and brawny and having a mustache and beard.

All the couples participating in AID group sessions felt relieved that the secrecy surrounding their infertility had been discarded and that they could discuss mutual problems and fantasies with each other. Greater openness in this respect will promote equality between partners and increase public acceptance of AID as a form of treatment.

Unexplained infertility

In approximately 15% of investigated couples infertility investigations reveal no abnormalities. A highly frustrating situation then arises for both the gynecologist and the couple. For both sides it is impossible to explain, and difficult to accept the failure to conceive in the absence of abnormalities. There is considerable ambivalence in this situation. On the one hand, it is disappointing for the doctor not to be able to say: 'I have found the cause of your problem and will institute treatment'; on the other hand, there is some relief for the couple that no major obstacle to conception is evident and yet frustration that a pregnancy that is physically possible fails to occur.

Unexplained infertility in apparently physically normal couples is sometimes assumed to be psychogenic in nature. Infertility has been described as 'psychic conflicts sailing under a gynecological flag' (Menninger, 1943). Several writers have referred in various ways to infertility: as a somatic symptom representing unconscious protection against post-partum psychosis; as a psychosomatic defence against feared pregnancy and motherhood; as a somatic response to intrapersonal stress; and as a basic flaw in the self which provides narcissistic injury and unjustifiable hurt. To date no satisfactory explanation has emerged as to why the uterus and reproductive system are singled out as the channel for expression of such intrapersonal conflicts.

The major theory frequently proposed as explanatory has a psychodynamic basis. Psychodynamic theory views infertility as a woman's unconscious rejection of pregnancy, childbirth and motherhood. One hypothesis is that this rejection arises from fears of coitus, which may be identified as a female equivalent to male castration fears, and culminates in a belief that birth will mean destruction of self. Another hypothesis with a social role emphasis is that the infertile woman has a learned identification with a hostile, rejecting mother and that this has resulted in the development of serious conflicts within the daughter's sexuality and femininity. She has grown up with deep-seated feelings of personal inferiority and resentment of men. Fears of loss of love and approval which would produce uncomfortable feelings are of necessity repressed and replaced with demands on the self for perfection in all things and, in particular, to be the 'perfect wife and woman' who must, therefore, become a mother. Within this framework, the real self is subjugated to, and replaced with, a martyr image of well-meaning, indirect, uncomplaining altruism which has traditionally been regarded as the feminine stereotype. The supposed effect of the conflict between desire and fear is inhibition of one or more of the mechanisms necessary for conception. Alternatively, such factors may operate during pregnancy. Vanden Burgh *et al.* (1966) reported that after suture of the cervical os for repeated abortion, five out of nine women developed a post-partum psychosis and three others had psychotherapy before carrying to term. Another source of conflict has been suggested for the woman with a strong intellectual drive who has been unable to resolve the choice between an ambitious and competitive career and that of domesticity and motherhood. Conflicts would also be expected when the husband is treated as a son. Parenthood may then become a threat to the couple's close relationship. Conception may be avoided by a process of unconscious collusion. These types of conflicts may exist in various combinations. Associated sexual dysfunction may be present.

There are many single case study reports in the psychoanalytic literature which link the occurrence of pregnancy with resolution of such conflicts. Psychodynamic theory may well be an appropriate framework in which to understand the occurrence of infertility in some couples.

Rubenstein (1951) used psychotherapy to make unconscious feelings conscious and to gain understanding of conflict about pregnancy. Four out of five of Rubenstein's patients became pregnant. More recently Sarrell and De Cherney (1985) randomly allocated twenty couples with a history of secondary infertility with no detectable organic etiology to two treatment groups. In one group each couple was seen by a psychotherapist. Psychodynamic techniques were used in the 2-hour interview to uncover previously unrecognized psychological conflict and psychodynamic interpretation was offered. The most prevalent conflicts found were problems between the woman and her mother in which psychological boundaries between the two women were confused, sexual problems, marital discord, and fear of pregnancy. The second group of ten couples was not seen by the psychotherapist. At follow-up eighteen months later, six of the ten women in couples interviewed by the psychotherapist had become pregnant. The findings of this exploratory study suggest that brief psychotherapeutic intervention might be helpful in enhancing reproductive potential. The mechanism by which fertility was enhanced was not clear. Sex counselling at the time of interview appeared to help reverse sexual dysfunction present in the seven couples. It is possible that resolution of pregnancy-related conflicts may have affected physiological factors in the neurotransmitter pathways and thereby enhanced reproductive potential.

Mai *et al.* (1972) suggested that three criteria were necessary for the diagnosis of psychogenic infertility: the couple must be involuntarily childless in the sense of engaging in coitus with the expressed intention of producing a child; there must nevertheless be clear evidence of reluctance to become a parent in one or both partners, with interview data corroborated by developmental history; and there must be a clearly defined mechanism whereby conception is prevented despite the stated desire to conceive. These criteria were met by only two of the fifty infertile couples studied by Mai *et al*. The mechanism was behavioural in each case: failure to ejaculate and an unexplained preference for intercourse during menstruation, respectively. The authors noted that some suggested psychosomatic mechanisms might be difficult to demonstrate with current methods of investigation. Bos and Cleghorn (1958) have postulated various ways in which fertility could be impaired by autonomic pathway links to the genital tract. These included chemical changes of a spermicidal nature in the vagina, interference with implantation in the endometrium, and spasm of the Fallopian tubes. Conclusive proof in the individual is hard to imagine. As Mai (1969) emphasized, the presence of blocked tubes in an infertile woman of disturbed personality cannot be taken to imply a psychogenic connection.

Humphrey (1984) warns that to diagnose a psychological cause of childlessness by a process of exclusion would be unwarranted, and unless there are strong indications such as the criteria proposed by Mai *et al.* (1972) the couple should be given the benefit of any doubt. A further reason for caution is that techniques for investigating infertility are still being developed and may ultimately reveal pathology in some of the unexplained infertility couples. Humphrey (1984) therefore suggests that with the available evidence fertility should be regarded as a biological variable, the expression of which might be modified by social and emotional factors. One example of how this may occur is via emotional effects on the hypothalamic-pituitary-ovarian pathway. Many patients with infertility have disordered hormonal production, either subtly or grossly. Steroidal hormonal messengers have also been shown to influence mood and sexual behaviour. As noted earlier, both the diagnosis and treatment of infertility are inherently stressful. Anxiety and depression produced might affect hormonal pathways which themselves might then exacerbate both infertility and the distress of the individual.

IN-VITRO FERTILIZATION

Couples arrive at the IVF clinic after many years of investigations and operations and often a long waiting list. Many have not faced the personal meaning of childlessness, as they keep hoping for a successful outcome of the next procedure. IVF is thus the end of the infertility career path. The procedure itself is highly stressful, involving repeated blood sampling and medicalization of what is usually the most intimate aspect of a couple's relationship. Both members of the couple are expected to 'perform'. The male is expected to produce semen when required, rather than ejaculation occurring spontaneously in response to erotic stimulation. The woman is expected to ovulate and to become pregnant once the embryo has been implanted. Failure of any of these events to occur after so much emotional, physical and financial expense can lead to feelings of failure in one or both of the infertile couple. Further, as IVF is regarded as 'the end of the road' for infertility treatment, when pregnancy does not occur (and this is the most likely outcome for the majority of participants) the couples are often forced to really face the concept of infertility for the first time. This can trigger a crisis, which if successfully resolved can lead to an adaptation to infertility. Thus the clinician involved with IVF needs to be aware of the role that psychological factors might play in the etiology, modification and sequelae of, and adaptation to infertility.

The achievement of pregnancy

As already mentioned, the objective of both the gynecologist and the infertile couple is the achievement of a successful pregnancy. If this goal is reached, the result is of course highly rewarding for both parties. In our experience, however, the occurrence of conception, especially in cases of long-standing childlessness, is not always received with the joy and enthusiasm that could be expected. Sometimes the news 'You are pregnant' is received with some reservation or even dislike and depressive feelings. These feelings may be caused by an initial unwillingness to believe the good news out of fear that it might not be true or that something might go wrong with the pregnancy.

Some couples pursue pregnancy desperately, partly under the influence of social pressures. The actual knowledge of being pregnant confronts them with the inevitable consequence of this pregnancy: the coming of a child. They suddenly realize that, unconsciously, they have separated their wish to *achieve* a long-desired result (pregnancy) and the real wish to nurture and bring up a child. Quite often they have adapted their social situation and their own relationship to a life without children, and this situation might well be disturbed by a potential intruder, however much the latter has been wanted.

These negative feelings, which usually are of transient nature, can be very confusing for both the couple and the gynecologist, because they are felt as incomprehensible ingratitude and lead to guilt feelings on the one side and irritation on the other. Still, they should be considered as a very natural reaction and not as emotional instability. They represent part of an adaptation process to cope with a completely new situation, and should be met with understanding and empathy.

Failure to achieve pregnancy

When pregnancy is not achieved despite a long and thorough investigation and intensive treatment, a frustrating situation for both gynecologist and patient is again created, which often, because of pressure by the couple, leads to an endless reiteration of diagnostic tests and unnecessary additional treatment. Women are operated on over and over again and couples travel from one doctor to another, unnecessarily prolonging their own torment. Although it is difficult to resist such pressures, it should also be said that it is often the doctor who, unwilling to accept his failure to perform, keeps the couple on this infertility merry-go-round.

There comes a moment at which one should honestly ask the question: 'Who really wants the baby, the doctor or the patient?' It should be realized that the painful working-through of the various phases of the mourning process after infertility is established can only take place adequately if an end has been made to all diagnostic and therapeutic interventions. This decision should be taken with sufficient determination to withstand the couple's natural urge to continue. The gynecologist should overcome his own frustration, admit his inability, and direct his attention and energy to helping the couple to cope with their grief. Sometimes it is less painful to endure a negative certitude than a positive incertitude.

IMPLICATIONS FOR THE CLINICIAN

It is evident that psychological issues are intimately intertwined with organic processes. Psychological factors may exacerbate or diminish infertility and affect the couple's adaptation to both diagnosis and treatment. There is a clear need for the gynecologist to avoid the simple dichotomy of physical versus psychological and to be aware of the role played by psychological and social factors. By doing so he may be able to help couples to have a more comfortable passage through infertility investigations and treatments and promote their successful adaptation to the result of the programmes. Psychiatrist, psychologist and social worker should be members of the infertility team, available to see referrals and to facilitate the work of the gynecologist. Attention to the following can improve the doctor-patient relationship and help the gynecologist to determine when referral to the psycho-social team is indicated.

Gynecologist-couple interaction

Much of the foregoing concerns the emotional relationship between a gynecologist and an infertile couple. It should be kept in mind that this relationship has two specific aspects: in the first place, the gynecologist is (at least in our society) usually a male, and, secondly, he usually already has what the couple are seeking: a family. This situation can influence the gynecologist's attitude towards the problems confronting the couple.

The male physician's attitude to his female patient will to a great extent be determined by his attitude to women in general. If the doctor sees a woman as someone whose main function is to serve and reproduce, his feelings of superiority — already present in any doctor-patient relationship — will be intensified. Under these conditions the patient will be less likely than ever to talk about her real problems, especially if they are concerned with sexuality or are relational in nature. Thus, the position of the male physician relative to his female patient is characterized by a double sense of superiority: the unavoidable superiority of the physician in relation to his patient, reinforced by the traditional superiority of men in relation to women. This combination produces the classic picture of the male physician: paternalistic and sympathetic but stand-offish. He knows what is good for the patient and is not influenced by emotions. These characteristics are not necessarily bad and in some situations can even be valuable. But they are not sufficient to generate adequate communication and can therefore constitute an obstacle to a real understanding of the patient's problems. They lead to what might be called one-way traffic: talking, advising and prescribing predominate, leaving little space for listening, understanding and empathy.

There is still another aspect of the relationship between gynecologist and patient that deserves special attention. The woman who is the patient of a male physician will often adopt a passive, accepting, and dependent attitude, and this will not promote communication between them, either. In this context one of the important functions of the gynecologist should be to encourage the female patient to be verbal and independent and thus greatly increase not only ability to express her real feelings but also the degree of her involvement in the investigation and the treatment.

Is the foregoing applicable to the relationship between the male gynecologist and the infertile couple? Acceptance of the proposed model of interaction in relation to an infertile couple has the following advantages:

1. An equally divided sense of solidarity towards both partners.

2. A better awareness and understanding of the psycho-social consequences of female infertility.
3. A better awareness and understanding of the psychosexual consequences of male infertility.
4. Avoidance of a 'father-daughter'-like relationship with the female patient, especially by enhancement of her sense of responsibility and self-esteem.
5. Avoidance or at least understanding and handling of the some times associated feelings of jealousy in the male partner towards the doctor, who is seen as responsible for a pregnancy. 'Doctor, I am so grateful to you; this is in fact your child.'
6. Last but not least, an easier acceptance of failure of success by putting into proper proportions the social pressures to have a family and by endorsing the emancipation of both men and women in the way described above.

Interview the couple

Infertility is always a problem of the couple. No matter whether one or both are shown to have a problem, the other partner also has a very strong interest in investigation and treatment. Involving both from the outset would seem to be optimal for both the couple and the clinician. From the couple's point of view, there may be less anxiety when they see the doctor together. With raised courage they may be more likely to ask about their fears and concerns and are more likely to remember jointly the information later.

The doctor has the opportunity to discuss with the couple their expectations to share the staff's awareness that the programme will add to their stress, and to explore the motivations and mixed feelings of each partner. The doctor also has a unique chance to observe how the couple interact and whether there are any relationship problems which might be exacerbated by the treatment. The couple can be reassured that infertility itself has no deleterious effects on sexual functioning, but informed that many couples find their sexual relationship impaired by the meaning of the diagnosis or by the many treatment demands on what should be a spontaneous activity. If a couple have sexual problems they should be offered sex counselling with a member of the clinic team. The clinician should begin to prepare the couple for a non-pregnant outcome. By sharing with the couple the impact that this often has, he may help the couple to start to face this eventuality.

In addition to providing information about the organic aspects of infertility, the doctor can inform the couple of the importance of psychological preparations for the procedure ahead. These may include attendance at patient self-support groups, stress reduction techniques such as relaxation classes, and regular discussions with a member of the psycho-social team for support before, during and after the procedure.

The management plan should be developed with the couple, the gynecologist discussing the various investigation and treatment options with them. The exact sequence and pace of tests and treatment should be negotiable. The price of such tests and treatments should also be considered.

Individual assessment

It is of course necessary to see each member of the couple individually for both physical and psychological assessment. From the psychological viewpoint the clinician should identify those patients likely to be at risk psychiatrically who might benefit from early referral to the psycho-social team. These would include patients with a current psychiatric disorder or past psychiatric treatment, those where there is concern about motivation, stability of the marriage and capacity for parenthood, and those with unrealistic expectations of the treatment. Berger (1977) recommends referral of those patients with unexplained infertility. The results of our pilot study suggest these patients may be more at risk. The following factors may also indicate vulnerability of the patient to stress: lack of confiding relationships; significant life stress in the previous year; use of immature, neurotic or psychotic coping strategies; a history of separations from family members during development; loss of a parent before the age of 11; previous depression following a loss; and family history of psychiatric disorders.

The individual interview also provides the clinician with the opportunity to explore the patient's fears, guilt and shame about infertility and allows the patient to discuss privately any sexual or marital concerns.

Counselling

It is stongly recommended that one member of the infertility team with training in counselling should be assigned to each at-risk couple. The couple should see the counsellor before embarking on any procedures, particularly IVF. The couple should then be seen during the work-up, during the in-patient phase and afterwards for weekly follow-up until the counsellor discharges the patient. By the counsellor seeing the patient prior to the procedure it is hoped that a relationship will be established which will enable counsellor and couple to work together to deal with the stress and crisis which may result after IVF. Some couples will need more help than others. It is recommended that such attendance should be an integral part of the IVF programme. The experience so far is that when counselling has been on a purely voluntary basis few patients have utilized these services adequately. As relationships were not established pre-IVF, patients failed to return when distressed after the failure of IVF.

The counsellor may come from the disciplines of general practice, nursing, psychology or social work but should work under the broad supervision of the team psychiatrist. Other roles of the psycho-social team are to conduct stress reduction groups, facilitate patient support groups and staff support groups, and provide community and doctor education programmes.

There are many possible outcomes following participation in infertility programmes. A number of women become pregnant. As this has occurred after many years of frustration, the couple may be understandably anxious about the pregnancy, delivery and parenthood. Continuation of counselling during the pregnancy and immediate post-partum may be of great assistance in enabling many of these couples to make a smooth transition to parenthood.

Some couples who do not succeed in pregnancy at their first attempt at treatment enrol again in the treatment programme and appear to deal with their disappointment by their new hopes. Many couples suddenly confront the full enormity of the meaning of their infertility when the miracle pregnancy has failed to occur. This may produce a state of crisis or disequilibrium. Such crises are usually time-limited and push towards resolution. The outcome may take one of three possibilities. The person may emerge from the crisis with the same level of functioning as previously; the person may emerge from the crisis with increased strength and emotional insight; or the person may regress to a less stable mode of functioning. A positive side to the disequilibrium is that since existing coping mechanisms have failed the person is open to change and growth. If the arousal of the person in crisis can be focused upon a tangible problem, the skilled therapist can help the individual to resolution and adaptation. Many affects may be manifest, including those of anger, guilt, anxiety, depression and grief. Recognition of sterility represents many losses: of children; of genetic and family continuity; of fertility and what that implies to sexuality; and of the pregnancy experience itself. It is of course difficult for many couples to grieve over infertility while there is still uncertainty about the permanency of loss. This must especially apply to those couples whose infertility is unexplained.

The role of the therapist is to support the couple through the difficult process of confronting their infertility and the alternatives. Assisting the person through the grief process requires that each difficult feeling be recognized, worked through and overcome. Such feelings may be reactivated in the future at times of crises or anniversaries but if adequately dealt with are not likely to be as overwhelming or severe. Successful resolution leads to a gradual sense of perspective in which infertility is put in its proper place in life and the individual begins to plan a future life again.

CONCLUSION

The role of psychological factors in infertility is complex. Psychological issues intertwine with the physical, often with additive effects. The very diagnosis of infertility is likely to cause stress. In addition, the many investigations and procedures may have compounded distress. There are probably a small number of patients in whom psychological factors may induce infertility, but in the majority psychological factors may exacerbate infertility and influence the patient and partner's response. Mental, sexual, marital and social adjustment may all be affected. The procedure of IVF is likely to have a further impact.

The clinician is advised to incorporate consideration of the psychological aspects of infertility into every aspect of the investigation and treatment programme. The addition of a psycho-social team can assist the gynecologist in this and help the couple to make an optimal adjustment.

REFERENCES AND FURTHER READING

Benedek, T. (1952). Infertility as a psychosomatic defence. *Fertil. Steril.*, **3**, 6, 527–37

Berger, D. M. (1977). The role of the psychiatrist in a reproductive biology clinic. *Fertil. Steril.*, **28**, 141–5

Bos, C. and Cleghorn, R. A. (1958). Psychogenic sterility. *Fertil. Steril.*, **9**, 84–98

Humphrey, M. (1984). Infertility and alternative parenting. In

Broome, A. and Wallace, L. (eds) *Psychology and Gynaecological Problems*, pp 77–94. Tavistock Publications, London

Mai, F. M. M. (1969). Psychiatric and interpersonal factors in infertility. *Aust. NZ J. Psychiat.*, **3**, 31–6

Mai, F., Munday, R. and Rump, E. (1972). Psychiatric interview comparisons between infertile and fertile couples. *Psychomat. Med.*, **34**, 430

Menninger, K. (1943). Emotional factors in organic gynaecologic conditions. *Bull. Menninger Clinic*, **7**, 47–55

Morse, C. and Dennerstein, L. (1985). Infertile couples entering an *in-vitro* fertilisation programme — a preliminary survey. *J. Psychosomat. Obstet. Gynaecol.*, **4**, 207–19

Platt, J., Fischer, I. and Silver, M. (1973). Infertile couples: personality traits and self-ideal concepts discrepancies. *Fertil. Steril.*, **24**, 972–6

Rubenstein, B. B. (1951). An emotional factor in infertility. *Fertil. Steril.*, **2**, 1, 80–6

Sandler, B. (1961). Infertility of emotional origin. *J. Obstet. Gynaecol. Br. Commonwealth*, **68**, 809–15

Sandler, B. (1968). Emotional stress and infertility. *J. Psychosomat. Res.*, **12**, 51

Sarrel, P. M. and De Cherney, A. H. (1985). Psychotherapeutic intervention for treatment of couples with secondary infertility. *Fertil. Steril.*, **43**, 897–900

Vanden Burgh, R. L., Taylor, E. S. and Drose, V. (1966). Emotional illness in habitual aborters following suturing of the incompetent cervical os. *Psychosomat. Med.*, **28**, 257–63

Chapter 7

Chronic Pelvic Pain

INTRODUCTION

Pelvic pain is one of the most frequent complaints of women referred to gynecologists. The term 'chronic pelvic pain' is used to describe pain which has been present for more than six months. The management of the chronic pelvic pain patient is recognized as difficult and frustrating for both gynecologist and patient. The extent of the problem is revealed by the following comments in the literature: 'one of the most difficult challenges in gynecological practice'; 'one of the most perplexing problems facing the gynecologist'; and that 'premature resort to surgery is the characteristic error in the present day treatment of these patients with pelvic pain'. Such comments suggest that at least some of the problems encountered might reflect attempts by gynecologists to treat pain as a purely somatic event until proved otherwise. Yet pain is ultimately always a psychological event. In order for pain to be experienced from a peripheral stimulus, not only must peripheral pain nerves and neuraxis be intact but the input must be processed psychologically by the central nervous system. For example, a woman in a comatose state is not aware of pain from a fractured pelvis.

Pain has many possible meanings and may be thought of as a universal language expressing discomfort or suffering via the body. Sooner or later everybody suffers great pain or shares another's pain. Early theories of pain reflected the specificity theory. This held that there were specific pain fibres and that the degree of pain perception was proportional to the degree of tissue damage caused by a noxious stimulus. Increasing evidence that psychological factors such as anxiety, personality, and social variables can influence the perception of painful stimuli favour a model of pain in which noxious input from the periphery is modulated by descending influences from the brain. The gate control theory of pain proposed by Melzack and Wall (1965) provides an anatomical basis for the interaction of ascending and descending influences in the spinal cord. Whilst the model is imperfect in the view of some researchers, it has established the principle of pain perception as the result of multiple influences, both at the spinal cord and the cerebral level. Such a view means that the relationship between noxious stimuli and pain intensity will not be linear. Thus psychological or social factors may result in minimal pain complaints despite the presence of major trauma. Conversely, psychological variables may result in severe complaints of pain when there is objective evidence of only minimal trauma.

Pain as a sensation has three major components. These are the sensory qualities (burning, pricking, stabbing), the suffering qualities (distressing, tiring) and the behaviours resulting from the pain, such as avoiding certain activities. In such a multi-dimensional model of pain all pain is real, but the amount of activity in each of the systems may not be equal. The importance of the distinction between the sensory and the suffering components of pain is illustrated by both narcotic administration and prefrontal lobotomy, both of which appear to diminish mainly the suffering dimension. The patient remains aware of the subjective experience of 'hurt' but is no longer distressed. Psychologists have also emphasized the distinction between the behaviours accompanying acute and chronic pain. Acute pain is typically associated with increased anxiety and autonomic arousal. Chronic pain may be associated with behaviour similar to that of depression, with loss of appetite, sleep disturbance, and social withdrawal.

With an understanding of the historical development of the meaning of pain, etiological mechanisms of chronic pelvic pain are now considered.

ETIOLOGY

Organic

Chronic organic conditions which may contribute to a pain problem are classified in Table 4 (adapted from Renaer and Guzinski, 1978). Non-gynecological causes will not be further discussed here, although it is assumed that care will be taken to exclude such causes by utilizing appropriate diagnostic techniques.

Table 4 Organic causes of pelvic pain

Non-gynecological
Gastro-intestinal: irritable bowel syndrome, diverticulitis, Crohn's disease, cancer of sigmoid colon, appendicitis

Orthopedic: hyperlordosis, spondyloarthrosis of the lumbar area, prolapsed disc, abdominal wall neuralgia

Urological: cystitis, ureteral stones, ptosis of a kidney with obstruction of urinary flow

Gynecological
Episodic
Trauma or infection of urethra/vagina
Dyspareunia due to vaginismus
Mittleschmerz (mid-cycle pain)
Dysmenorrhea
Adenomyosis
Endometriosis

Continuous
With anatomic abnormalities: chronic infection with tubal dilation, residual ovary syndrome, pelvic tumours, genital prolapse, endometriosis, adhesions

Without anatomic abnormalities: chronic pelvic pain syndrome, pelvic congestion syndrome, Allen-Masters syndrome, spastische parametropathie, pelipathia vegetativa, pelvic sympathetic syndrome, pelvic neurodystonia, broad ligament neuritis

Whilst pain from chronic pelvic inflammatory disease and gross ovarian endometriosis is readily understandable, there is much controversy about the significance of adhesions and of the various syndromes associated with chronic pelvic pain.

Adhesions

There is much contention in the surgical literature about whether adhesions cause pain. Some women are observed to have massive adhesions without experiencing pain whereas others experience intense pain with mininal adhesions. Such findings have led some clinicians to conclude that adhesions in themselves may not be enough to cause pain. Therapy for adhesions has been limited and results have often been disappointing. Conservative methods have included bowel regulation with vegetable bulk laxatives, hot baths, local heat and rectal diathermy. Recent animal research suggests that high molecular-weight dextran solutions, alone or in combination with steroids and antihistamines, may be effective in preventing adhesion formation. Outcome studies of similar compounds in humans are needed to determine both if such compounds are effective in preventing re-formation of adhesions after surgical division, and any effects on pain perception.

Chronic pelvic pain syndromes

These syndromes variously named have an ill-defined pathogenesis and less than satisfactory treatment. Symptomatology in them is similarly described as lower abdominal or iliac fossa pain, worsened premenstrually or by physical activity, sometimes with low back pain, often with deep dyspareunia, and includes leucorrhea, menstrual disturbances, constipation, depression and anxiety. Most patients are married and between 20 and 40 years of age. On examination the uterus and adnexa may be tender and there may be tenderness of the posterior parametrium. The pathogenesis suggested for such complaints has varied. Allen and Masters (1955) ascribed the syndrome to laceration of uterine ligaments with acute uterine retroversion. Spasm of broad ligaments and pelvic nervous over-activity are other suggested mechanisms. Histological abnormalities such as inflammation or immuno-allergic processes have also been suggested. One of the most popular explanations has been that of circulatory abnormalities resulting in pelvic varicosities.

In evaluating the evidence for such disorders it is apparent that these syndromes were described prior to the development of modern diagnostic techniques such as laparoscopy. Even with such techniques the significance of many so-called abnormalities with regard to the pathogenesis of pain is not known. It is also possible that disease processes may be present but remain undetected because current investigative techniques are not sensitive enough to detect certain pathological processes.

Renaer (1980) investigated with laparoscopy women with chronic pelvic pain and a control group of infertile women without pain. Of the fifty-four pain patients nineteen had endometriosis and seven had sequelae of acute salpingitis. In twelve the cause of the pain was not clear, and sixteen were found to have chronic pelvic pain without any obvious pathology. No tears of the uterosacral ligaments were found. Although some depressions were found in the broad ligament the significance of these is not known. Renaer (1980) also investigated the role of the paracervical tissues in chronic pelvic pain. No evidence for spasm of the broad ligament was found. Pathological examination of the cervix and posterior parametrium in a sub-group of chronic pain patients and non-pain controls found no difference histologically between the two groups.

This study also considered the role of circulatory disturbances. The pelvic congestion syndrome is said to result in hyperemia of the uterus, sometimes with resultant hypertrophy, pelvic varicosities and an increase in pelvic transudate. Renaer found no uterine hyperemia. Varicosities were observed. When parity and use of steroids were controlled for, there was no difference in the frequency of varicosities between non-pain controls, chronic pain patients with endometriosis and chronic pain patients without obvious pathology. The latter group did have significantly more peritoneal fluid present at operation.

Phlebography has been used by other investigators to study pelvic circulation. There appears to be some evidence that pelvic circulation may be disturbed in at least some patients without other explanation for pelvic pain (e.g. Vermeersch et al., 1971). A review of pelvic phlebography studies reveals that while many pelvic pain patients show radiological signs of pelvic congestion so too do some patients who do not complain of pain.

Further studies are needed to clarify the role of circulatory factors in pelvic pain. Taylor (1950) has suggested that pelvic pain may be caused by vascular changes occurring in response to stress. Duncan and Taylor (1952) used a thermal conductance measure to study pelvic blood flow in ten chronic pain patients during an interview. Emotionally laden topics appeared to cause increases in blood flow, which returned to normal when neutral topics were discussed. A non-patient control group was not used so it is not known whether such changes are specific to pelvic pain patients. Recent psychophysiological studies of vaginal blood flow have found that normally sexually active orgasmic women show increases in vaginal blood flow only in response to sexual stimuli and not with anger or anxiety. Further research is needed to confirm Duncan and Taylor's findings, perhaps utilizing the methodological advances in the measurement of pelvic blood flow in sexual arousal.

In summarizing the role of organic factors in the genesis of pelvic pain it should be noted that many recent studies utilizing laparoscopy have found no obvious pathology present in a large proportion of the women studied. Gillibrand (1981) found that of 331 women presenting with pelvic pain only 37% had any identifiable pathology present at laparoscopy. Murphy and Fliegner (1981) studied twenty-two women diagnosed as having pelvic inflammatory disease and were able to confirm the diagnosis in only seven. These findings highlight the difficulty for gynecologists in diagnosing the source of pelvic pain, a difficulty which appears to be shared by general surgeons with regard to abdominal pain. Two studies have shown that a large proportion of women who undergo appendicectomy for acute abdominal pain are found to have normal appendices at biopsy (Creed, 1981; Crossley, 1982).

Psychological

Observations that many chronic pelvic pain patients had no demonstrable organic pathology or insufficient pathology to account for symptoms has led to interest in psychological factors. Subsequent findings which have led to increased consideration of psychological factors include the seemingly high incidence of psychopathology in such patients, poor response to organic approaches to the treatment of pain and experimental research on factors influencing pain perception.

There are many possible mechanisms by which psychological factors could cause or potentiate pain. Psychoanalytic theories suggested that pelvic pain could represent a displacement from other problems, such as sexual conflicts and concerns about femininity and childbearing. In some the pain mechanism was said to arise from a hysterical conversion reaction. It is interesting in this regard to note that pain was a prominent feature in the four women that Freud described in his essays on hyseria. Engel (1981) referred to certain individuals as pain-prone patients, predisposed by early developmental factors to exploit pain as a psychological means of adaptation later in life. The pain symptom was said to appear whenever an unconscious need to suffer remained unsatisfied, as in situations of real or threatened loss or where strong forbidden sexual or aggressive sensations cause guilt. The pain site was determined by the history of the patient's object relations and the kind of conflict. In pelvic pain, psychosexual conflicts were said to predominate. Other psychogenic explanations for pain include the (uncommon) hallucination of pain in psychotic states such as schizophrenia and severe depression. Pain of many types is a common symptom in psychiatric populations, suggesting a possible lowering of the pain threshold in such patients. It may reflect increased muscle tension, this also arising from psychological causes. The work of Duncan and Taylor (1952) suggests that emotions can influence pelvic blood flow, leading to long-standing pelvic circulatory changes and pain. The importance of social factors is strikingly illustrated by the occurrence of the Couvade syndrome, in which fathers act as if suffering from pains during or after their wives' childbirths.

Other psycho-social explanations derive from experimental studies of pain. Those studies relevant to the problem of chronic pelvic pain were reviewed by Pearce and Beard (1984). An important variable is the individual's expectation of pain. When subjects were given instructions which raised their expectations of experiencing pain, they were more likely to describe pain than when no mention of pain was provided in their instructions. Thus patients who have already experienced pelvic pain might have a lower threshold for perceiving pain subsequently. Such a factor might be important in maintaining chronicity of pain. Pearce and Beard (1984) also highlighted studies demonstrating that predictability and control over pain may influence pain perception. Both behavioural control, the belief that one can do something to decrease pain, and cognitive control have been shown to increase pain tolerance. Cognitive control is the belief that cognitive strategies, such as pleasant imagery and relaxation techniques, can be used to control distress. Most patients with chronic pelvic pain feel they have little control over the pain. Psychological techniques which promote feelings of control over pain are likely to be helpful in increasing pain tolerance. These techniques are listed in Figure 3. Anxiety is a further variable which has been shown experimentally to influence pain perception. Chronic pain populations tend to have high levels of anxiety. Relaxation techniques have proved helpful in reducing both anxiety and perceived intensity of pain. Social factors have also been shown experimentally to influence pain perception. These include both modelling effects and the way in which the behaviour of others, such as a spouse, might reinforce pain behaviours.

Many studies have sought to determine whether pelvic pain patients

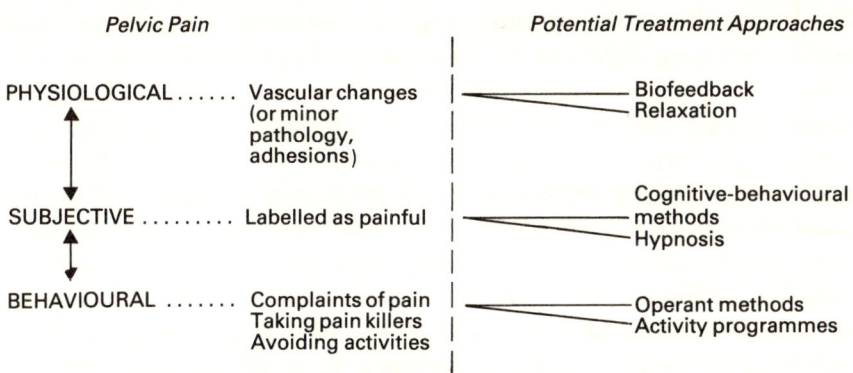

Figure 3 Psychological therapies for chronic pelvic pain.
(From Pearce and Beard, 1984)

without obvious organic pathology differ psychologically from those with demonstrable pathology or from those without pain. The research has been beset by many methodological problems. These were reviewed by Reading (1982), who highlighted the lack of homogeneity in sample groups, the questionable reliability of the method used to determine whether organic pathology was present, the lack of appropriate statistical analysis using multivariate techniques, and the degree to which the patients studied could be considered representative of patients with chronic pelvic pain.

A major problem has been the recognition that the occurrence of a correlation between certain psychological characteristics and pain does not imply causality. In fact, neuroticism, for example, has been shown to increase with the chronicity of the problem and to diminish as the pain responds to treatment. Early studies reported a high incidence of psychopathology among chronic pelvic pain patients of undiagnosed etiology. Gidro-Frank et al. (1960) found thirty-eight of forty such patients to have significant psychiatric disturbances: schizophrenia (four); borderline psychosis (ten); severe neurosis (twenty); moderate neurosis (three); mild neurosis (one). A major problem in this study is that only one of the control group of twenty-five pregnant patients was considered normal. Such findings suggest possible selection bias in the sample and that the method of psychiatric diagnostic procedure used may have been unreliable. Similar problems exist in a number of other studies.

Prill (1964) was among the first to note that a large percentage of patients (with pelipathia vegetativa) studied had no evidence of psychopathology. It was also noted that it was not possible to identify any specific sort of underlying psychological conflict or distress which characterized women without organic explanation for pelvic pain. Later studies utilizing laparoscopy to confirm diagnosis have found little association between pathology and psychiatric findings. That is, the incidence of psychiatric disorder was as high in the pathology group as it was in the group without organic pathology (Castelnuovo-Tedesco and Krout, 1970; Renaer et al., 1979; Rosenthal et al., 1984). Others such as Beard et al. (1977) found differences on psychometric testing (higher neuroticism scores), when women with and without demonstrable organic explanation for pain were compared. The groups were not matched for the chronicity of pain. The obvious possibility exists that being in pain for some time may induce psychological disturbance in the appropriately predisposed individual, regardless of the magnitude of any organic contributions to the problem.

In addition to findings of increased neuroticism in chronic pelvic pain patients, some studies report many sex-related problems amongst these patients. Beard *et al.* (1977) found that no-pathology pelvic pain patients rated themselves more negatively on a number of sex-related concepts. Once again the question of causality is dubious, as patients were not matched for chronicity of pain and the frequency of associated dyspareunia in such patients would be expected to contribute to sexual problems. Gross *et al.* (1980) found early traumatic sexual experiences (incest) in nine out of twenty-five patients with unexplained pelvic pain. They suggested that such experiences lead to anxieties in adulthood which unless resolved will be manifested as pelvic pain. No control data are available to determine how common such experiences are among the general population or other patient groups. Conflicting findings were reported by Petrucco and Harris (1982), who found 72% of their twenty-four women with unexplained pelvic pain were orgasmic and questionnaire scores indicated no sexual dysfunctions.

The role of stress in precipitation of pain was indicated by the study of Benson *et al.* (1959). The onset was attributed to stress factors in twenty-two out of thirty-five cases without demonstrable pathology. Selectivity of recall and the tendency to draw associations in order to establish explanations might bias such retrospective accounts. Studies suggesting an association between chronic pelvic pain and certain developmental disturbances, such as emotional deprivation and interpersonal difficulties extending back to childhood (Duncan and Taylor, 1952; Gross *et al.*, 1980), suffer from similar methodological flaws. In summary, while there is considerable evidence experimentally that psychological and social factors may contribute to the perception of pain, the role such factors play in the pathogenesis and maintenance of chronic pelvic pain has not been adequately delineated. What is apparent is that patients who suffer from chronic pelvic pain of whatever etiology have a high incidence of psychopathological traits. These may add to the patient's distress, lead to further difficulties in social functioning and serve to exacerbate or maintain the pain. There exists the possibility that current diagnostic methods may not be sensitive enough to reveal the etiology of pain in at least some of those without obvious organic pathology. Thus it seems wise to suggest a shift from the orientation adopted by many workers intent on proving psychogenic etiology to instead focusing on the role psychological and social factors may be playing in the patient's distress and in maintaining the disorder. Such an orientation has obvious implications for management.

MANAGEMENT

Recognition of the complex role of organic, psychological and social factors in pain perception and behaviours has led to the establishment of pelvic pain clinics with multi-disciplinary teams. These have the advantage that all factors can be assessed and appropriate treatment strategies devised. Many gynecologists have commented that referral to psychiatric clinics is often met with hostility and resentment by the patient, who may feel rejected by her gynecologist, that her pain is not accepted as real, and that she is labelled as 'neurotic'. The presence of psychologists, psychiatrists and social workers in the pain clinic is more readily accepted by the patient as part of a total team approach to help her to better manage her pain. Gynecologists often find women suffering from chronic pelvic pain to be difficult management problems and appreciate the support engendered by the team structure. Principles of management are then as follows:

Education

An education programme about the complex nature of pain should commence when women first arrive at the clinic. The patient should be informed that no matter how her pain initially arose both physical and psychological factors are likely to be important in why it is still present. Thus a full assessment of physical, psychological, interpersonal and occupational functioning is necessary. This may involve a number of investigations and assessments by different members of the clinic team. The aim is not to establish a cause of, and thus abolish all pain. In chronic pain it is to be expected that the result of assessment will be a list of factors thought to be contributing to the maintenance of pain. Similarly, treatment may comprise a number of modalities all aimed at helping the patient to regain control over her pain. As the investigation is comprehensive and the problem complex, patients are to be discouraged from presenting to the emergency room or other gynecological clinics during treatment, and instead to bring their complaints to the pain clinic.

Simultaneous investigation

In order to establish the role of organic factors, radiological and surgical investigations may be needed. It is recommended that psycho-social assessment should proceed at the same time. This should include a full psychosomatic history (see Chapter 1). Special attention to sexual history will be needed because of the frequent occurrence of sexual problems. A special aspect of history-taking is to discover the meaning of the pain to the patient. Cancer fears are often prominent in these women and the fear itself and its relationship to the pain must be dealt with openly. Psychometric testing should not be used to establish a diagnosis but rather to supplement clinical findings with details of specific deficit areas. The object of psychological assessment is thus to obtain a full understanding of the patient rather than to merely seek a psychogenic explanation for pain. Particularly helpful may be the keeping of a pain diary. This should include daily accounts of the frequency and intensity of any pain and associated behaviours, such as medication use or activity reduction. At subsequent visits details of possible precipitants or reinforcers of pain can be sought and the patient encouraged to be aware of these and incorporate them in the diary. The diary thus evolves into a behavioural analysis.

The usefulness of such an approach is illustrated by the way in which negative findings at laparotomy are received by the patient. Confrontation with the information that there is nothing organically wrong may lead to denial and rejection of this information. Patient response is likely to be quite different with education in the philosophy of pain as being caused and maintained by multiple factors. Investigation of all aspects simultaneously allows an explanation of the pain to gradually evolve.

Involvement of partner/family

It is recommended that the woman's partner, or, where appropriate, other significant persons, be involved from the outset. This serves several functions. Education about the nature of pain, the clinic programme and the expectations of the therapy makes it less likely that family members will obstruct therapy. A pertinent history about the patient can be obtained, which may help to reveal reinforcers of pain behaviours and the effects of the pain on interpersonal relationships. The partner may subsequently be asked to help in treatment strategies, for example to take part in sexual counselling or to help to reinforce 'well behaviours'.

Treatment strategies

Therapies will be drawn from the different disciplines represented at the clinic and an individual approach devised for each patient, depending on the factors thought to be important from the assessment. Physical approaches may include surgery, where warranted, and the use of a pain 'cocktail', in which the proportion of analgesic is progressively reduced. Psychotropic drugs may be needed where major psychiatric disorder is present. Psychological aspects of patient care will vary from simple measures such as education and reassurance to the use of specific therapy techniques such as those of biofeedback or hypnosis. As many women with chronic pelvic pain have been described as alexithymic or as having difficulties in expressing feelings, part of the treatment strategy may be directed at helping them to develop such abilities so that distress does not have to be somatized. Rosenthal *et al.* (1984) noted that over-reaction to minor discomfort was a common problem amongst the women they studied. As time went by, their patients learned to notice exacerbation of pain due to stress. Clinic visits were used sometimes for brief supportive psychotherapy, crisis intervention, and continuing education about the connection between psychological and physical well-being. O'Neill (1958) reported that the two most valuable techniques were what amounted to discussion to determine the sources of anxiety, friction and discontent, and relaxation therapy. Two prospective studies have shown that a substantial reduction in the number of attacks of pelvic pain can be achieved by relatively simple psychotherapy (Beard *et al.*, 1977; Pearce *et al.*, 1981). It is not clear what form of psychotherapy is most effective. Sexual counselling should be considered when sexual problems are evident.

The model suggested by Pearce and Beard (1984) (see Figure 3) is helpful in illustrating the way in which psychological factors can be utilized in chronic pelvic pain. Few of the treatment strategies suggested have been evaluated for chronic pelvic pain. However, their utility in other chronic pain problems suggests an application. There are anecdotal reports of relaxation training being useful for women with undiagnosed chronic pelvic pain (Beard *et al.*, 1977; Petrucco and Harris, 1982; Pearce *et al.*, 1982).

CONCLUSION

Utilizing a model of pain perception and management which recognizes the influence of multiple factors should reduce frustrations for both gynecologist and patient. While some patients will be found to have organic pathology of a degree which accounts for the level of distress, many have only minimal pathology — the significance of which is still contentious. These patients were often diagnosed as suffering from one of the chronic pelvic pain syndromes, such as pelvic congestion. Our lack of knowledge of the significant pathogenesis in such cases suggests a diagnosis of 'chronic pelvic pain without obvious pathology' may be preferable to assigning the name of a syndrome, which implies a certain etiological mechanism.

Experimental studies have demonstrated the profound influences on pain perception of psychological and social factors. Clinical studies have found a high incidence of psychopathology in pelvic pain patients. Accompanying sexual problems are frequent. Psycho-social factors may exacerbate or maintain pain in many patients. These powerful factors can also be used positively to help the patient to adapt to the pain. In order to utilize them the clinician must from the outset adopt a psychosomatic approach. The patient's re-education about the nature of pain and the role of multiple factors in causation and treatment should begin at the first visit. Multi-disciplinary clinics probably provide the optimal way to investigate and manage these problems.

REFERENCES

Allen, W. M. and Masters, W. M. (1955). *Am. J. Obstet. Gynecol.*, **70**, 500

Beard, R. W., Belsey, E. M. and Lieberman, J. C. M. (1977). Pelvic pain in women. *Am. J. Obstet. Gynecol.*, **128**, 566–70

Benson, R., Hanson, K. and Matarazzo, J. (1959). Atypical pelvic pain in women: gynecologic psychiatric considerations. *Am. J. Obstet. Gynecol.*, **77**, 806–23

Castelnuovo-Tedesco, P. and Krout, B. M. (1970). Psychosomatic aspects of chronic pelvic pain. *Int. J. Psychiat. Med.*, **1**, 109–26

Creed, F. (1981). Life events and appendicectomy. *Lancet*, ii, 1381–5

Crossley, R. B. (1982). Hospital admissions for abdominal pain in childhood. *J. Royal Soc. Med.*, **75**, 772–6

Duncan, C. H. and Taylor, H. C. (1952). A psychosomatic study of pelvic congestion. *Am. J. Obstet. Gynecol.*, **64**, 1–12

Engel, G. L. (1981). *Medicina Psicomatica e Sviluppo Psicologico*. Cappelli Editore, Bologna

Gidro-Frank, L., Gordon, T. and Taylor, H. C. (1960). Pelvic pain and female identity. *Am. J. Obstet. Gynecol.*, **79**, 1184–202

Gillibrand, P. N. (1981). The investigation of pelvic pain. Communication at the Scientific Meeting on *Chronic Pelvic Pain — a Gynaecological Headache*, Royal College of Obstetrics and Gynaecology, May, London

Gross, R. J., Doer, H., Galdirola, D., Guzinski, G. and Ripley, H. S. (1980). Borderline syndrome and incest in chronic pain patients. *Int. J. Psychiat. Med.*, **10**, 79–86

Melzack, R. and Wall, P. D. (1965). Pain mechanisms: a new theory. *Science*, **150**, 971–9

Murphy, A. and Fliegner, J. (1981). Diagnostic laparoscopy: its role in the management of acute pelvic pain. *Med. J. Aust.*, **1**, 571–3

O'Neill, D. (1958). Tension pain in gynaecological practice. *J. Obstet. Gynaecol. Br. Emp.*, **65**, 106–9

Pearce, S., Knight, C. and Beard, R. W. (1981). Pelvic pain — a common gynaecological problem. In van Hall, E. V. and Bos, G. (eds) *Psychosomatische Verloskunde en Gynaecology* (Boerhaave Cahiers No. 3), pp 97–106. Stafeus Wetenschappelijke Uitgeversmaatschapi B.V., Holland

Pearce, S., Knight, C. and Beard, R. W. (1982). Pelvic pain — a common gynaecological problem. *J. Psychsomat. Obstet. Gynaecol.*, **1**, 12

Pearce, S. and Beard, R. W. (1984). Chronic pelvic pain. In Broome, A. and Wallace, L. (eds) *Psychology and Gynaecological Problems*, pp 95–116. Tavistock Publications, London

Petrucco, O. M. and Harris, R. D. (1982). A Psychological and venographic study of women presenting with non-organic pelvic pain. Paper presented at the *8th New Zealand Congress*, Auckland, New Zealand

Prill, H. J. (1954). *Psychosomatische Gynakologie*. Urban and Schwarzenberg, Munich and Berlin

Reading, A. E. (1982–83). A critical analysis of psychological factors in the management and treatment of chronic pelvic pain. *Int. J. Psychiat. Med.*, **12**, 129–39

Renaer, M. (1980). Chronic pelvic pain without obvious pathology in women. *Eur. J. Obstet. Gynecol. Reprod. Biol.*, **10/6**, 415–63

Renaer, M. and Guzinski, G. M. (1978). Pain in gynecologic practice. *Pain*, **5**, 305–31

Renaer, M., Verbommen, H., Nijs, P., Wagemans, L. and van Hemelrijck, T. (1979). Psychological aspects of chronic pelvic pain in women. *Am. J. Obstet. Gynecol.*, **134**, 75–80

Rosenthal, R. H., Ling, F. W., Rosenthal, T. L. and McNeely, S. G. (1984). Chronic pelvic pain: psychological factors and laparoscopic findings. *Psychosomatics*, **25**, 833–8

Versmeersch, A., Claus, P. and Leeart, C. (1971). Technique sequentielle d'hysterophlebographie par voie endo-uterine. *Gynecol. Obstet.*, **70**, 589–607

Chapter 8

Hysterectomy

INTRODUCTION

Gynecological surgery poses a unique stress for women because of the identification of the reproductive organs both with sexuality and with the wider concept of feminine identity. This stress is particularly apparent when one considers surgery such as hysterectomy, which produces loss of both the monthly 'badge' of femininity (menses) and the important female role of childbearing.

Matters of concern for the gynecologist have included the increasing frequency of this operation and the long-reputed association with psychological and sexual sequelae. Research findings in this area have often appeared contradictory. It is helpful to examine first the meaning of hysterectomy in a historical perspective.

HISTORICAL THEMES

Throughout the history of medicine the uterus has been a focus of interest. The Egyptians, as indicated in the Kahan Papyrus (2000 BC), saw the uterus as having an important and powerful effect on mental life. This theme formed the basis for the hypothesis that removal of the uterus will also have a profound emotional effect. In the absence of anatomical knowledge — surprising in itself because the Egyptians mummified their dead — the uterus was conceptualized as an independent creature capable of wandering about at will within the body of its host. These wanderings of the uterus were said to cause various morbid symptoms, and a number of methods were devised for attracting it back to its rightful place.

The second historical theme was related to the concept that fertilization and childbearing were needed to produce uterine gratification, with consequent emotional stability. This theme occurred in a later Egyptian papyrus, and was expanded by Hippocrates and Plato. Hippocrates prescribed marriage for older virgins and widows who suffered from what he termed 'suffocation of the womb'. In the *Timaeus*, Plato wrote: 'The womb is an animal which longs to generate children. When it remains barren too long after puberty it is distressed and sorely disturbed, and straying about the body and cutting off the breath . . . brings the sufferer into the extremest anguish and promotes all manner of disease besides.' This theme seems to underlie psychoanalytic views on feminine sexuality as being passive, masochistic and dependent on childbearing ability.

A third theme concerned the importance of personality characteristics in the woman's adaptation to her uterus. Aretacus of Cappadocia, a Greek physician of around 200 AD, suggested that younger, flightier women were more vulnerable to afflictions of the uterus. Recent prospective studies have investigated the effects of premorbid psychological functioning on outcome after hysterectomy.

Historically, vaginal hysterectomies seem to have been performed successfully for prolapsed gangrenous uteri from at least the time of Soranus (100 AD). One of the earliest reports of adverse sequelae was that made by a Venetian professor, Giacomo Berengario da Carpi (1480–1550), who recorded that his father had removed the gangrenous uterus of a patient. She lived for many years afterwards and resumed sexual relations with her husband, but experienced little sexual satisfaction.

The last century saw the development of anesthesia and techniques which made abdominal and vaginal surgery possible. Nevertheless, only a year after the coining of the term 'hysterectomy' Von Krafft-Ebing observed that psychosis followed hysterectomy more frequently than it did other surgical procedures. Hysterectomy is now one of the most frequently performed major operations in women and concern about the psychological aspects of the procedure has continued.

FREQUENCY OF HYSTERECTOMY

The frequency of hysterectomy in many countries is so high that women are now being encouraged by health insurance firms to seek a second opinion before agreeing to it. In Australia it was estimated that 40% of insured women in the 20–25 years cohort could expect to have a hysterectomy in their lifetime. In the Netherlands the incidence of hysterectomy per 1000 women of all ages rose from 2.9 to 3.9 during the 1970s. This compared with 6.5 in 1979 in the United States, where over 50% of women were expected to have a hysterectomy.

Hysterectomy may be performed for organic causes. However, in many women there is no demonstrable pathology.

Table 5 gives a survey of the changes, in the Netherlands, in the frequency of the various indications relative to each other. The decrease of uterine myoma as indication for hysterectomy is striking. It is possible (and to be hoped) that it reflects a more conservative attitude to uterine myoma. It is also conceivable that the relative decrease of this indication is to be ascribed to a decrease of the mean age of the whole group of hysterectomized women due to other indications at younger ages.

Another striking finding is the relative and absolute increase of indications 3 and 4, both of which may be considered to some degree disputable. This holds particularly for 'inflammation and other affections of the uterus', a diagnosis which is seldom arrived at pre-operatively and is almost always made retrospectively as a histological diagnosis (cervitis, endometritis) without clinical significance. The number of hysterectomies performed on these indications rose between 1974 and 1979 by as much as 64%.

Group 5 comprises mainly medical indications (infections, benign and malignant tumours) and has shown little or no change in frequency in the course of this period, with the exception of the equally debatable indication 'abdominal pain, pain in the genital organs', which showed an absolute increase amounting to 49% between 1974 and 1979.

Table 5 Indications for hysterectomy in the Netherlands

	1974/1975		1978/1979		Absolute rise 1974–1979
	Absolute	%	Absolute	%	%
1. Leiomyoma of the uterus	7.880	36	7.872	30	0
2. Disorders of menstruation	5.169	24	6.093	23	18
3. Prolapse of uterus or vagina	2.754	13	4.168	16	51
4. Inflammations and other affections of the uterus (excluding tumours)	1.688	8	2.767	11	64
5. Others	4.321	19	5.472	20	27
	21.812	100	26.372	100	21

Source: Netherlands Central Bureau of Statistics (Diagnosestatistiek Ziekenhuizen)

Table 6 Frequency of hysterectomy in different departments in the Netherlands (according to annual reports for 1980)

	Admissions	New patients	Hysterectomies	Hysterectomies/new patients
U 1	2806	4001	79	51
U 2	2979	3817	153	25
NU 1	3479	4267	149	29
NU 2	3329	3600	479	8

U = University department; NU = Non-university department

Table 7 Frequency of hysterectomy in different departments in the Netherlands (according to annual reports for 1980)

	Diagnostic curettage	Hysterectomy	% vaginal hysterectomies	Hysterectomies/ diagnostic curettages
U 1	233	76	40	0.34
U 2	333	153	45	0.46
NU 1	254	149	55	0.59
NU 2	482	479	75	0.99

U = University department; NU = Non-university department

Tables 6 and 7 show the frequencies of hysterectomy and diagnostic curettage in two university and two non-academic teaching hospitals in the Netherlands, arranged to facilitate comparison, in relation to the total number of admissions and new patients per year. The data are taken from the annual reports for 1980 of the hospitals in question. It is evident from these figures that there are great differences in the frequency of hysterectomy between hospitals with comparable patient material. According to the annual reports, these differences cannot be explained by differences in the frequency of vaginal prolapse or prolapse of the uterus, and it may therefore be assumed that the indications for hysterectomy differ widely between hospitals.

Causes suggested for the considerable increase in the number of hysterectomies performed annually in the Netherlands include an increase in the female population. This group is estimated to have increased there by 7% between 1971 and 1979. It seems probable that in this period there has been a slight shift in the age distribution toward older ages, but this would not explain an increase of 44% in the frequency of hysterectomy.

Another possible reason includes menstruation-related complaints (see Table 5). It may be that an increase in these is related to an increase in smoking and drinking alcohol as these habits are associated with menstrual complaints. It is also possible that women in the Western world may now perceive as abnormal menstrual blood loss and/or discomfort which would previously have been tolerated. A possible reason for this lowered tolerance of menstruation may have been a long-term use of the oral contraceptive pill, which usually produces a marked reduction in the amount of bleeding and discomfort experienced. Women are often advised to cease taking the pill after the age of 35 and to use other forms of contraception. Some women then find the return to 'normal' menstruation intolerable.

Of major interest is that when women complain of heavy periods this does not necessarily mean heavy blood loss. Prolonged heavy blood loss would lead to anemia and ill-health, and hysterectomy is justifiable to prevent this. When women who complained of heavy periods were studied, only 50% actually showed evidence of increased blood loss and only a much smaller percentage were anemic. Blood might comprise only 20% of the total fluid content of menstruation and yet it is this component that is so important in determining therapy. The number of sanitary pads or tampons used bears little or no relationship to the actual amount of blood loss (Fraser, 1981).

Other factors also influence the amount of blood loss. For example, in many primitive societies menstrual flow is scanty and usually lasts only one day. Nutrition may be an important factor. It is important to reflect that regular menstruation is an artefact of modern society. In more primitive societies the menarche or first period occurred later and the menopause earlier, and pregnancy and prolonged breast feeding (with associated lack of periods) occupied much of the interim period.

In an evolutionary sense we have not had time for our bodies to adjust to the tremendous changes wrought by our modern contraception technology. This may be a major reason for women in Western countries expressing dissatisfaction with their periods and seeking hysterectomy. There are now medications available which help to reduce the amount of bleeding and pain. These may not be acceptable to all patients or completely successful in eradicating symptoms.

Another major factor which can influence both the amount of menstrual blood loss and discomfort and the woman's tolerance of and perception of this is her emotional state. Studies in the UK (Gath, 1980), USA (Martin et al., 1977) and Australia (Ryan et al., 1983) have found an extraordinarily high number of women (55%, 57% and 47%) to be suffering from significant emotional illness pre-operatively. The incidence of such symptoms in the general population is only 12–14%. The main types of psychiatric problems suffered were those of depression and anxiety.

What do these findings mean? It is possible that at least some of these psychological problems represented anxiety about the forthcoming operation. In the UK study women may have been waiting to have the operation for some time. When it is known that the operation is needed a long wait can increase anxiety. Interestingly, over half of the patients with psychiatric problems had significantly improved when interviewed eighteen months post-operatively (Gath *et al.*, 1982).

Another major explanation of the presence pre-operatively of such large numbers of women with psychiatric problems is that women with psychological problems or some inner distress may present to doctors with gynecological symptoms. In our society negative attitudes to mental illness are common. Women with psychological distress may tend to present to their doctor saying 'I feel sick' rather than 'I feel sad or miserable or nervous'. Our whole medical system seems to encourage this focus on physical complaints rather than emotional ones. As one of our patients remarked after hysterectomy, 'I go to the doctor when I feel bad, but I always seem to get the wrong thing', by which she meant operations instead of treatment of her emotional problems. It is well known that when people do feel depressed or anxious they often focus on bodily symptoms and tend to perceive these more negatively.

Lastly, it is possible that psychiatric problems may adversely influence the menstrual cycle.

Gynecologists obviously have a major influence on the rate of hysterectomy as they must make the final recommendation that such an operation is necessary. In making a diagnosis the gynecologist relies on the description of the illness provided by the patient and examination of the patient. Yet, as already described, it may be unrealistic to expect women to be accurate reporters of such symptoms as blood loss. Availability may also be important. There are more gynecologists per head of population in both Australia and North America than in the United Kingdom, which has a lower hysterectomy rate (of practising gynecologists). In the Netherlands the number increased by 33% in the period in question, but since the total number of other gynecological operations (excluding sterilization) decreased rather than increased in this period (see above), the role of this factor in the phenomenon is not clear.

There is no doubt that some doctors and some patients are more surgically orientated, whilst others are more drug orientated. Some women have the operation as an alternative to sterilization, particularly if they wish to stop menstruation.

It is obviously important for the clinician to be aware of the factors which may be influencing the pathway to hysterectomy, in making a decision about whether hysterectomy is indicated for an individual woman.

PSYCHOLOGICAL AND SEXUAL SEQUELAE AFTER HYSTERECTOMY

Conceptual studies

Early writers such as Deutsch (1944) and Drellich and Bieber (1958) emphasized loss of childbearing capacity in terms of women's feminine self-concepts.

Although Deutsch did not make a particular study of the effects of hysterectomy, her major work, *The Psychology of Women*, seems to have been regarded by several writers as the definitive statement on women's psychosexual development. Using classical psychoanalytic theory, she emphasized not only the instinctual nature of feminine passivity, masochism, and narcissism, but also motherhood and the potential for motherhood as the ultimate expression of sexuality in women: 'When a woman has ended her existence as bearer of a further life she has reached her natural end — her partial death — as a servant of the species.' In terms of this biologically based theory, the uterus figured importantly in a woman's psychological life. Self-esteem was derived from the fulfilment of biological function. The loss of childbearing capacity adversely affected the self-concept of femininity. For Deutsch, the concept of femininity had no social or cultural overtones.

Drellich and Bieber (1958), as part of their wider research on the psychological impact of cancer surgery, made a more detailed study of the perceived importance of the uterus to women who were to undergo hysterectomy, and the subsequent adjustment to the new state. For this study it was assumed that the individual's adaptive techniques become obvious under stress (included by the removal of the uterus); existing defences may not be able to deal with the stress; previously unformulated attitudes and conflicts may find conscious expression, beliefs and attitudes about the organ at risk may come to the surface; and lastly, that behaviour patterns emerging after surgical removal of the organ may indicate the specific role that the organ played in the psychological economy.

The patients in this study were twenty-three randomly selected pre-menopausal women, all of whom had undergone a total hysterectomy and bilateral salpingo-oophorectomy. Nine of them had a malignant disease of the uterus. The women were interviewed pre-operatively and post-operatively during convalescence and at six and twelve months. The pre-operative interviews were focused on the patient's conscious attitude and emotional response to the impending surgery and loss of the uterus. In the post-operative period adjustment on the sexual and social levels was explored. The study brings to our attention the variety of ideas women have about the value and function of their uterus and how these may reflect the woman's general pattern of adaptation. The chief pre-operative concern of the women was the loss of childbearing capacity, but the ability to have children did not have the same meaning for all the women. For example, for some the child was to provide a general sense of gratification, while others wanted to have children to please their husband. Two patients in the group who already had large families welcomed the operation which would relieve them of contraceptive worries. Contrary to expectation, the majority of women in the study regarded menstruation as a necessary and valuable function, again for various reasons. The women were also concerned that the operation would affect sexual response.

Drellich and Bieber (1958) interpreted their findings as showing how intimately the uterus was related to the concept of femininity and that its loss was experienced as damaging to femaleness. They suggested that the psychoanalytic concept of 'castration anxiety' should extend, beyond anxiety pertaining to the male genital organ, to include the uterus.

Crisis theory

Early writers, e.g., Lindemann (1941), and later Drellich and Bieber (1958) described hysterectomy as being a uniquely traumatic experience for many women. More recently, the crisis nature of hysterectomy has been emphasized and the process of adjustment to the stresses involved has been explored. Raphael (1972) described the crisis of hysterectomy along the parameters of certain functions theoretically critical to crisis resolution; namely, affective, defensive, cognitive, and reality aspects and object relations. Raphael theorized that within these areas women would experience some interactions that would be useful for crisis resolution whilst others would be unhelpful.

One hundred married women aged between 20 and 47, who underwent hysterectomy for a non-malignant condition, were interviewed between the seventh and twelfth post-operative days. The matched control group comprised cholecystectomy patients. A questionnaire study (1974) assessed the outcome after thirteen months for 85% of the patients. Only 38.8% of these women described themselves as having no health impairment; 24.7% suffered substantial impairment; and the remainder some impairment. There was a significant difference between the hysterectomy and control groups in the areas of depression and other general symptomatology. Of the parameters associated with poor outcome, the degree of non-support in the social network was found to be the most potent force. The women also expressed the need to be able to ventilate feelings of annoyance and apprehension about the operation and to be given explanations.

The crisis theory offered a useful approach, since it allowed for consideration of the intrapsychic aspect of the individual in relation to the crisis event, as well as the interaction with environmental factors, the dynamics of which require consideration for effective intervention to take place.

Another study (Kaltreider *et al.*, 1979) which explored the process of adjustment to hysterectomy was based on the hypothesis that a common phase of adjustment follows traumatic events. There is initially a blocking-out or avoidance of the realization of the traumatic event (denial), followed by gradual admittance to consciousness. In this manner the trauma is gradually accepted, together with its accompanying discomfort. If the trauma is not worked through in this manner, the patient may become symptomatic in a fashion described as the Stress Response Syndrome.

Kaltreider and co-workers interviewed twenty-eight women twelve months after hysterectomy. Only 38% had adjusted successfully to the operation, the Stress Response Syndrome being present to a mild degree in 43% of the group and to a severe degree in 18%. Those women who had not coped with the operation were more likely to see themselves as having deteriorated sexual functioning or felt themselves to be changed as women. Women who had shown a pattern of poor adjustment to previous losses were at risk for the development of severe Stress Response Syndrome. This study provided a useful description of the phasic pattern of adjustment.

Methodology

Both retrospective and prospective studies have investigated the outcome of hysterectomy. It is difficult to interpret the results, because the criteria for the evaluation of outcome varied from extremes such as admission to a mental institution to such vague notions as 'emotional disturbance'. In some studies hysterectomy was associated with oophorectomy, and some samples included patients with both benign and malignant lesions. Sample size differed greatly, and the method of data collection varied from interviews to questionnaires and analysis of the medical and psychiatric history. Some studies did not include sufficient details about the sample or results.

Comparisons between results obtained in different countries and different samples are limited by the influence of cultural factors on a woman's perceptions about, and the values she places on, her uterus, differences in psychiatric criteria between countries, and differences in the systems of health care between countries, which may determine the woman's pathway to surgery and her experience of hysterectomy — in other words her interaction with the health-care system. Nevertheless, a review of the literature yields interesting information, as follows.

Retrospective studies

These studies were performed to test the hypothesis that, because of the symbolic significance of the uterus, hysterectomy could be followed by a higher incidence of psychological and sexual disorders. Several authors found evidence of adverse psychological or sexual sequelae, i.e., an increased psychiatric-hospital admission rate compared with other surgery or with expected community rates (the most frequent diagnosis was depression); an increased incidence of psychiatric referral (especially for depression); an increased frequency of treatment with antidepressants in a general-practitioner setting; and deterioration of the sexual functioning of many patients after hysterectomy.

Meikle et al. (1979) quoted eight studies which failed to find adverse consequences of hysterectomy. In three of these studies there was an increased incidence of adverse sequelae. Munday and Cox (1967) reported that 33⅓% of their sample reported emotional distress. Bragg (1965) found the risk for psychiatric-hospital admission to be slightly greater after hysterectomy than after cholecystectomy, although the difference was not statistically significant. Patterson and Craig (1963) studied one hundred psychiatric in-patients who had undergone hysterectomy. As only 15% were admitted in the first year after hysterectomy, these authors concluded that the hysterectomy itself was not a particularly stressful experience. The other studies cited by Meikle suffered from many methodological difficulties, including failure to report the method or measures used and high attrition rates. One author reported that he 'interrogated' his patients.

In the study of Dennerstein et al. (1977) sexual relationships were found to have deteriorated in thirty-three women (37%), thirty women (34%) stated that their sexual relationships had improved since the operation and twenty-six (29%) detected no change. The sexual morbidity incidence found was higher than that of 28% obtained in an earlier Australian study (Munday and Cox, 1967), but was similar to that of 38% found in a controlled study of general practice patients (Richards, 1974). Rather than focusing on the frequency of such sequelae, subjects were studied to determine which factors were associated with a poor sexual outcome.

The following factors were of interest with regard to sexual dysfunction. When estrogens were not prescribed or were taken only sporadically, significantly more dyspareunia was found than when estrogens were taken continuously. The presence of remembered pre-operative anxiety concerning possible deterioration of sexual performance was associated with an overall deterioration of sexual functioning after the operation. There was a significant relationship between the presence of this type of pre-operative anxiety and subsequent loss of desire for sexual intercourse and increased dyspareunia. These results support a multifactorial etiology of the sexual dysfunction found.

Retrospective studies cannot yield conclusive evidence as to whether there are adverse sequelae of hysterectomy, because they cannot provide us with information about the patient's psychological and sexual wellbeing before the operation. Prospective design is needed to provide conclusive evidence of the effects of hysterectomy.

Prospective studies

Early prospective studies were mainly exploratory and descriptive, with little quantitative data or statistical analysis in the reports. Lindemann (1941) did include a control group and a careful examination of past and current psychiatric status, but he failed to indicate how many of his small sample had undergone hysterectomy. These studies did, however, identify risk factors for poor outcome.

Barglow (1964) compared the outcome after hysterectomy with that after tubal ligation. Since the women studied had neither actively sought sterilization nor had a choice of surgical procedure, it is hardly surprising that there was a worse outcome for the more final operation of hysterectomy.

Chynoweth (1973) and Raphael (1974) investigated the general health outcome and sexual response after hysterectomy. Both reports suffer from brevity, which makes it difficult to follow the method used. Apparently, the same tests were not applied pre- and post-operatively, so the evaluation of health impairment became rather subjective, with little more validity than that reached by retrospective studies. Furthermore, although both chief investigators were psychiatrists, no mention is made of the psychiatric health of patients pre-operatively.

In three studies, no significant change in the parameters studied was found after hysterectomy. The same measures were used pre- and post-operatively, but the duration of follow-up was probably too short (three to six months) in view of the many studies which suggest that the process of adjustment to hysterectomy may take twelve to twenty-four months. One of these studies (Barglow, 1964) had a 42% drop-out rate, probably reflecting the technique of leaving rating scales with the patients for completion and return.

The recent studies of Martin *et al.* (1977, 1980) and Gath (1980; *et al.*, 1982) are of considerable interest. Both utilized intensive psychiatric interviews and psychological rating scales both pre- and post-operatively. There are some interesting similarities and differences between these studies. Different criteria for psychiatric illness were used and different rating scales. The investigators also differed: in the case of Martin *et al.* there was a male psychiatrist in a hospital setting, while Gath utilized female social workers and psychologists who visited the patients in their own homes.

Prior to the operation, both study populations had extremely similar incidences of psychiatric illness (55–57%). The type of diagnosis varied. This may reflect real differences in the women studied or their pathways to surgery. For example, the British women had to wait for surgery and may have been understandably more anxious by the time of operation. Since the hysterectomy rate in the USA is twice that of the UK, it is possible that more women with Briquet's Syndrome are operated on in the USA. Alternatively, the difference in type of diagnosis might simply reflect the different criteria used. The Present State Examination used by Gath has no separate category recognizing Briquet's Syndrome (a somatization disorder). In a recent prospective study by the present authors (Ryan et al., 1983) a high rate of psychiatric morbidity pre-operatively was also found. This study investigated thirty women prior to hysterectomy, using the Present State Examination as a measure of psychological health, and also sought to identify Briquet's Syndrome, using Feighner's criteria. Only one woman in the sample received this diagnosis, in contrast to 27% in the Martin et al. study. In the latter study, of thirty-four women with sexual partners, eleven reported an increase in sexual intercourse post-operatively, nineteen reported no change and four (13%) reported a decrease.

The study of Gath, Cooper and Day (1982) asked women to rate the frequency and enjoyment of sexual intercourse on a five-point scale. 80% of women had recovered their pre-operative level of sexual activity by the fourth post-operative month. Six months after operation the reported frequency of intercourse was increased in 56% of patients, unchanged in 27% and decreased in 17%. Reported enjoyment of intercourse was increased in 39%, unchanged in 41% and reduced in 20% of women. Eighteen months after operation the findings were unchanged. As the sexual relationships of many of these patients must presumably have already been impaired by gynecological disorders prior to the hysterectomy, it is disappointing that so many failed to improve or worsened after the operation.

In summary, it would appear that the operation of hysterectomy adversely affects the sexual behaviour of some women. Oophorectomy in pre-menopausal women without adequate hormone replacement therapy is likely to have additional effects. The etiology of the effects of hysterectomy and bilateral oophorectomy is likely to be multifactorial.

Psychological factors such as the symbolic meaning of the uterus and/or ovaries to the woman, her previous adaptation, and her expectations of surgery are all important. Biological factors must also be considered. Masters and Johnson (1966) noted that the orgasmic contractions by muscles in the outer third of the vagina were accompanied by rhythmic contractions of the uterus. Zussman et al. (1981) noted that 'for some women, the quality of orgasm is diminished when these structures are removed'. Removal of ovaries additionally removes the gonadal hormones estrogen, progesterone and androgens. Asch and Greenblatt (1977) have established that both pre-menopausal and post-menopausal ovaries produce significant quantities of androgens, perhaps as high as 50%.

Few attempts have been made to directly correlate hormone levels with behavioural changes. Chakravarti *et al.* (1977) studied endocrine changes and symptomatology after oophorectomy in a hundred premenopausal women. They concluded that: 'The known changes in the concentration of circulating steroids cannot be related directly to the occurrence of symptoms in individual patients, neither to the level of gonadotrophins, until more information is available on the biologically active functions of the circulating hormones and on their interactions with other factors.' The possible role played by hormonal depletion may be studied by examination of clinical trials of hormone replacement therapy (see Chapter 10).

The recent prospective studies raise some interesting hypotheses. It would seem that the incidence of development of new psychiatric problems is small and that most psychiatric problems will occur in those who had psychiatric problems pre-operatively. It is interesting to speculate whether this has always been the case or is perhaps a reflection of the tremendous social changes of the past few decades: the de-emphasis of reproduction for women's self-esteem and the increase in women's knowledge about their bodies as well as their more active participation in their interaction with doctors. The two recent British studies of Gath *et al.* (1982) and Coppen *et al.* (1981) further suggest that the support provided by trial interviews may even have decreased the psychiatric morbidity in patients. This has obvious implications for the prevention of psychological sequelae.

CLINICAL IMPLICATIONS

How can the clinician lessen the likelihood of sequelae and help women to successfully adapt to surgery?

Pre-operative management

Psychological preparation should be carried out routinely in the same way as the patient is prepared for the physical aspects of the operation. Extra time or care may be needed with patients identified as being at risk of a poor outcome. The major risk factor for a poor outcome after hysterectomy is the presence of psychiatric morbidity before the operation, as revealed by interview, personality rating scales and a history of previous referral to a psychiatrist.

A summary of risk factors identified elsewhere in the literature suggests that other risk factors for a poor outcome will include: younger age (Raphael, 1974); lower educational status (Chynoweth, 1973); absence of any concern pre-operatively or excessive anxiety (Menzer *et al.*, 1957); absence of perceived support in the immediate social network (Raphael, 1974); poor relationship with mother (Chynoweth, 1973); and negative expecations of the operation (Dennerstein *et al.*, 1977).

The purpose of pre-operative preparation is to lessen anxiety about the possible effects of the surgery. This is best achieved in a supportive, empathic relationship where the patient is encouraged to discuss her feelings about the operation and to relate what she may have heard from others about the effects of hysterectomy. An educative approach by the doctor will help to dispel anxiety based on inadequate knowledge. Information on the anatomy and physiology of the reproductive system and genital organs, in simple language and illustrated by diagrams, is helpful to most patients. The nature of the operation, the reasons for it, and the expected changes can then be elaborated. Advice should be given on when normal activities, particularly sexual intercourse, can be resumed. As anxiety may limit the recall of information, this explanation might need to be repeated on several occasions or reinforced with a book suitable for women to read at home, such as *Hysterectomy: A Book to Help You Cope with the Physical and Emotional Aspects* (Dennerstein *et al.*, 1982). Where applicable, and if the partner is willing, it is desirable that he should be included in order to allay possible anxiety about the likely effects of hysterectomy and help him to understand the type of support his partner needs. Encouragement to discuss the operation is usually extremely beneficial. Ideally this should occur pre-operatively or, if this is not practicable, in the immediate post-operative period.

The value of pre-operative preparation was shown in an Israeli study which explored further the findings of Dennerstein *et al.* (1977) of an association between negative expectations of hysterectomy and sexual deterioration. Women in hospital undergoing hysterectomy were randomly assigned to a two-hour group discussion on hysterectomy or to the usual preparation by their gynecologist. The women who had attended the single group sessions were later found to be significantly better adjusted psychologically and sexually (Cohen *et al.*, 1981). This study demonstrates how even a minimum intervention of one session spent discussing the operation can have marked benefits for the patient.

Hormone therapy

Coppen *et al.* (1981) have demonstrated that estrogen therapy is of no benefit to pre-menopausal hysterectomized women with intact ovaries. Following bilateral oophorectomy or menopause, prophylactic hormone replacement therapy is indicated. In such patients estrogen administration will alleviate hot flushes, associated insomnia and fatigue and prevent dyspareunia due to atrophic vaginal changes. We have also found a beneficial effect of estrogen on mood and parameters of sexual response, such as sexual desire, enjoyment, vaginal lubrication and orgasmic frequency, in our studies of oophorectomized women (Dennerstein *et al.*, 1979, 1980). Other long-term benefits of estrogen replacement therapy must also be considered, such as the prevention of osteoporosis. Against the benefits of estrogen therapy must be balanced the risks, such as those of thrombo-embolism and exacerbation of diabetes or uterine cancer.

Follow-up

Therapeutic effects of follow-up interviews were suggested by the study of Coppen *et al.* (1981). Long-term follow-up by the family doctor or gynecologist will help to facilitate the adaptation to hysterectomy. This follow-up should continue for twelve months, as many problems may only become evident some months after surgery.

Therapy for post-hysterectomy depression

Psychiatric disorders occurring after hysterectomy should be evaluated and initially managed in the same way as disorders presenting at other times of life. A referred woman who is suffering from depression some months after hysterectomy should have a full psychiatric, mental state and physical examination performed.

The severity of the depression should be assessed and treatment of the depression begun accordingly. Any woman who is a suicide risk should be admitted to hospital. Women with moderate or severe depression are usually given antidepressants in the first place. When the depression is so severe as to be life-threatening or there has been no response to antidepressants, electro-convulsive therapy may be used. Hormone replacement therapy for those who have symptoms of hormone deficiency or have undergone bilateral oophorectomy may also be indicated. As the depression begins to improve, the clinician can begin to gently explore the significance of the operation to the patient. It is also important to evaluate the reactions of others significant in the patient's life.

Usually only supportive psychotherapy in combination with antidepressant medication is needed. Occasionally, a more intensive psychodynamically-orientated psychotherapy is needed when the operation has triggered severe conflicts in the patient.

CONCLUSION

In summary, what is evident from the accumulated research is that there is a great deal of psychiatric disturbance present before hysterectomy. Whilst most psychiatric and sexual problems after hysterectomy occur in women with pre-existing problems, some new cases also develop. Trial interviews may in themselves have been therapeutic for many women. The clinician has an important role to play: firstly, in determining whether hysterectomy is indeed the correct therapy and what the woman's emotional as well as physical response is likely to be; secondly, in adequately preparing a woman and her partner for the operation — psychologically as well as physically; and finally, in recognizing at an early stage women who are having difficulty adapting to the operation, and then arranging prompt psychotherapeutic intervention.

REFERENCES

Asch, R. H. and Greenblatt, R. (1977). Steroidogenesis in the postmenopausal ovary. *Clin. Obstet. Gynecol.*, **4**, 85

Barglow, P. (1964). Pseudocyesis and psychiatric sequelae of sterilization. *Arch. Gen. Psychiat.*, **2**, 571–80

Bragg, R. L. (1965). Risk of admission to mental hospital following hysterectomy or cholecystectomy. *Am. J. Pub. Health*, **5**, 1403–10

Chakravarti, S., Collins, W. P., Newton, J. R., Oram, D. H. and Studd, J. W. (1977). Endocrine changes and symptomatology after oophorectomy in premenopausal women. *Br. J. Obstet. Gynaecol.*, **84**, 767

Chynoweth, R. (1973). Psychological complication of hysterectomy. *Aust. NZ J. Psychiat.*, **7**, 102–4

Coppen, A., Bishop, M., Beard, R. J. et al. (1981). Hysterectomy, hormones and behaviour. A prospective study. *Lancet*, **1**, 126–8

Dennerstein, L., Wood, C. and Burrows, G. D. (1977). Sexual response following hysterectomy and oophorectomy. *Obstet. Gynecol.*, **49**, 92–6

Dennerstein, L., Burrows, G. D., Hyman, G. and Wood, C. (1979). Hormone therapy and affect. *Maturitas*, **1**, 247–59

Dennerstein, L., Burrows, G. D., Wood, C. and Hyman, G. (1980). Hormones and sexuality: effect of estrogen and progestogen. *Obstet. Gynecol.*, **56**, 3126–22

Dennerstein, L., Wood, C. and Burrows, G. D. (1982). *Hysterectomy: A Book to Help You Cope with the Physical and Emotional Aspects*, Oxford University Press, Melbourne

Deutsch, H. (1944). *The Psychology of Women*. Grune & Stratton, New York

Drellich, M. G. and Bieber, I. (1958). The psychological importance of the uterus and its functions. *J. Nerv. Dis.*, **126**, 322–36

Fraser, I. (1981). Perceptions of menstrual cycle symptomatology. In Dennerstein, L. and Burrows, G. D. (eds) *Obstetrics, Gynaecology and Psychiatry*, pp 97–104. York Press, Melbourne

Gath, D. (1980). Psychiatric aspects of hysterectomy. In Robins, L., Clayton, P. and Wing, J. (eds) *The Social Consequences of Psychiatric Illness*. Brunner Mazel Inc., New York

Gath, D., Cooper, P. and Day, A. (1982). Hysterectomy and psychiatric disorder: Levels of psychiatric morbidity before and after hysterectomy. *Br. J. Psychiat.*, **140**, 335–50

Kaltreider, N. B., Wallace, A. and Horowitz, M. J. (1979). A field study of the stress response syndrome. *J. Am. Med. Assoc.*, **242**, 1499–1503

Lindemann, E. (1941). Observations on psychiatric sequelae to surgical operations in women. *Am. J. Psychiat.*, **98**, 132–9

Martin, R. L., Roberts, W. V., Clayton, P. T. and Wetzel, R. (1977). Psychiatric illness and non-cancer hysterectomy. *Dis. Nerv. Syst.*, **38**, (12), 974–80

Martin, R. L., Roberts, W. V. and Clayton, P. J. (1980). Psychiatric status after hysterectomy. *J. Am. Med. Assoc.*, **244**, 350–3

Masters, W. H. and Johnson, V. E. (1966). *Human Sexual Response*. Little Brown, Boston

Meikle, S., Brody, H. and Pysh, F. (1979). An investigation of the psychological effects of hysterectomy. *J. Nerv. Ment. Dis.*, **164**, 36–41

Menzer, D., Morris, T., Gates, P. *et al.* (1957). Patterns of emotional recovery from hysterectomy. *Psychosomat. Med.*, **5**, 379–88

Munday, R. N. and Cox, L. W. (1967). Hysterectomy for benign lesions. *Med. J. Aust.*, **2**, 759–63

Patterson, R. M. and Craig, J. B. (1963). Misconceptions concerning the psychological effects of hysterectomy. *Am. J. Obstet. Gynecol.*, **85**, 104–11

Raphael, B. (1972). The crisis of hysterectomy. *Aust. NZ J. Psychiat.*, **6**, 106–15

Raphael, B. (1974). Parameters of health outcome following hysterectomy. *Am. J. Obstet. Gynecol.*, **118**, 417–24

Richards, D. H. (1974). A post-hysterectomy syndrome. *Lancet*, **ii**, 983–5

Ryan, M. M., Dennerstein, L. and Pepperell, R. (1983). Preoperative psychological and sexual adjustment in hysterectomy patients. In Burrows, G. D., Dennerstein, L. and Fraser, I. (eds) *Obstetrics, Gynaecology and Psychology*, pp 65–75. York Press, Melbourne

Zussman, L., Zussman, S., Sunley, R. and Bjornson, E. (1981). Sexual response after hysterectomy-oophorectomy: recent studies and reconsideration of psychogenesis. *Am. J. Obstet. Gynecol.*, **140**, 725–9

Chapter 9

Tubal Sterilization

INTRODUCTION

Tubal sterilization is one of the most frequently performed surgical operations. For the older woman it is the most popular method of contraception world-wide, and it is increasingly requested by young women of low parity who have completed their families. Sterilization differs from other methods in that it is difficult to reverse.

Doctor' attitudes to sterilization have changed greatly over the last two decades. Until the late 1960s the medical profession in many countries had lingering doubts as to the legality of sterilization performed for other than medical indications. The outcome for women who had sterilization performed for such reasons may have been influenced by their pre-existing health conditions, and by the absence of choice which sometimes existed precisely because of the nature of an existing health condition. Whilst women had consented to surgery, they may not have actively desired it, as would well-informed healthy women who conscientiously chose this as their preferred method of birth control. The values held in society today encourage, and indeed expect, women to make responsible decisions about family planning. Therefore, the attitudes of the medical profession which reflect these values have become correspondingly more positive.

Developments of medical technology which enabled sterilization to become a simpler and safer procedure have no doubt also been factors in increasing acceptability of the method to patients and their doctors.

Dissatisfaction with other forms of contraception may also have led to the increased demand for sterilization. For example, women who are over 35 years old and are overweight or who smoke heavily are often advised not to use the oral contraceptive pill. With the reduction in average family size, more women have completed their families at a younger age. There has been both a desire for permanent contraception and reluctance for prolonged use of some contraceptive methods.

Factors influencing the acceptability of tubal sterilization include the likely physical and psychological effects of the operation and the permanency of this method of contraception.

PHYSICAL SEQUELAE

There is increasing concern about possible adverse effects of tubal sterilization on menstruation. The incidence of menstrual disturbance following tubal ligation has been reported to vary from 25 to 60%. Possible reasons for such a discrepancy include those of research design (prospective *vs* retrospective studies), the response rate and the failure to control for effects of the previous contraceptive method. Kasonde and Bonnar (1976) collected objective evidence by measuring the blood loss in sanitary pads before and after sterilization and found no change at twelve months. Alder *et al.* (1981) controlled for previous contraceptive use and found that there was more change in menstrual patterns, both positive and negative, in sterilized women than in a control group of wives of vasectomized men. Two recent studies (Templeton and Cole, 1982; and Cooper, 1983) report an increased risk of hysterectomy for sterilized women. It is not clear whether the sterilization had adversely affected the women's menstrual patterns or whether their tolerance of menstruation had changed.

PSYCHOLOGICAL SEQUELAE

The rate of reported psychiatric morbidity has varied greatly. This contradictory situation also reflects methodological problems in research. In general, retrospective studies suggest a higher rate of psychiatric sequelae. The study by Enoch and Jones (1975) found at follow-up that 60% of the sample had suffered a psychiatric illness following the surgery. The high rate becomes understandable when one notes that only 34% had requested the surgery; the remaining women were 'advised' (by their doctors) to accept sterilization because of parity, marital problems, medical and/or psychiatric reasons. Those women who underwent surgery for the reason of high parity were more likely to have successful outcomes than those for whom other reasons were indicated. Another possible source of bias in this study is the diminished sample. One-third of the women invited to participate did not do so. Another study (Ansari and Francis, 1976) which found a high incidence of psychiatric sequelae reported that 51% of the sample of forty-nine considered their mental state to have deteriorated when they were interviewed six months after surgery. In this study one of the outcome parameters was the consumption of alcohol. 14% of the women reported increased alcohol intake at follow-up. Again, this was a mixed sample and those patients for whom high parity was the major reason for undergoing surgery had a better result. Personality factors were also found to affect outcome.

In contrast, Sim *et al.*(1973), in a retrospective study using a structured questionnaire, found that only 3.3% were adversely affected and previous psychiatric illness was not aggravated by the sterilization operation.

The most recent prospective studies, by Smith (1979) and Cooper *et al.* (1982), have the advantages of better methodology. Both arrive at conclusions quite different from the studies described above. In her Scottish study, Smith used Goldberg's Health Questionnaire and a standardized psychiatric interview to define psychiatric outcome for 196 consecutively referred women. At the initial pre-operative assessment, 25% of the women had scores indicating 'probable' caseness. Following sterilization these scores improved so that only 15% had scores in this range at the twelve months follow-up interview, when the attrition rate was 15%.

In their prospective study of women who had interval sterilization Cooper *et al.* (1982) interviewed women four weeks before, plus six and eighteen months after tubal ligation. Attrition rate was only 5.5%. The measure used for psychological outcome was the Present State Examination (PSE). The prevalence of psychiatric morbidity beforehand was 10.5%, which is no more than might be expected in the population. This was reduced to 4.7% at the six months interview and was 9.3% at the eighteen months post-operative follow-up interview. Only twelve people who were not 'cases' (as defined by the level of the PSE score) developed psychiatric symptoms at eighteen months. Conversely, fifteen of the twenty-one 'cases' beforehand had improved to become 'non-cases'.

Thus it would seem that the risks of psychiatric sequelae are small. There will, nevertheless, remain some women in whom such an operation is a factor precipitating psychiatric illness.

SEXUAL ADJUSTMENT

Once again, the results differ, with the recent prospective studies giving a more optimistic picture. Of the retrospective studies Ansari and Francis (1976) found that 78% of patients reported either no change or an improvement in their sexual relationships. Of the remainder, 22% reported that this aspect of their lives was negatively affected by surgery. Enoch and Jones (1975) found 44% to have improved sexual functioning, but 22% complained of loss of libido. 51% of those replying to Jackson's (1980) questionnaire in New Zealand reported their sexual life unchanged and 18% reported loss of libido. Cooper et al. (1982), in a prospective study, used a more objective measure of sexual adjustment. Patients were asked to report on frequency and enjoyment. Eighteen months after surgery, 28% of patients were reporting increased frequency, 26% decreased frequency, and for 46% this aspect remained unchanged. Enjoyment was increased in 22%, decreased in 6% and unchanged in 76%. There was a high correlation between psychiatric morbidity and psychosexual functioning at all interview phases. Smith (1979), in her prospective study, asked patients to rate sexual satisfaction on four points from very satisfactory to unsatisfactory. For 34% of the sample satisfaction was better, for 8% it was worse, and 58% reported no change. Neil et al. (1975) compared the sexual adjustment of women who had been sterilized with that of wives of vasectomized men. 54% of the sterilized women and 74% of the wives of vasectomized men reported a better sex life after the operation. Alder et al. (1981) also compared wives of vasectomized men with sterilized women. She found that wives of vasectomized men had a higher frequency of sexual intercourse, more were entirely satisfied with their sexual relationships and fewer had sexual problems.

In a summary of eight recent studies of sterilized women, Alder (1984) found that the majority of women report an improvement in their sex lives. This improvement was attributed by patients to removal of the fear of pregnancy and to greater spontaneity of sexual experiences. In a minority sexual satisfaction and frequency of sexual intercourse were reduced. Cliquet et al. (1981) reported that in most cases in which there was a deterioration there had been a pre-existing problem. Those who reported deterioration related it to post-operative complications, increased jealousy because of the fear of extra-marital relations, or difficulties in acceptance of demands from their partners for increased sexual activity. Most studies found no relationship between age, parity, length of marriage and post-sterilization sexual dissatisfaction.

DISSATISFACTION, REGRET AND REQUEST FOR REVERSAL

Regret is a difficult area to research as standardized measures may not give an accurate reflection of the patient's feelings. Estimates of regret vary. Schwyhart and Kutnar (1983) estimated that regret occurred in between 1 and 18%. Cooper et al. (1982) reported that 10.9% experienced regret, but only 3.1% would have considered reversal. Some women may regret the operation but on a rational basis acknowledge its necessity on realistic grounds, such as a medical condition which precludes other forms of contraception. Such women may report experiencing regret but would nevertheless take the same course of action again and do not consider reversal. For others regret may follow because the initial decision was hasty or uninformed or the situation which made sterilization seem desirable, e.g., a poor marital relationship or economic circumstances, may have changed. These women may then regret the earlier decision and may seek reversal. For these reasons, study findings relating to dissatisfaction or regret are not particularly helpful unless they specify reasons for regret.

Of particular interest are the reasons for request for reversal of sterilization. Lambert et al. (1984) divided such requests into two groups: those of women with a new relationship and those of women who have the same relationship as they had at the time of sterilization.

Request for reversal in a new relationship

The main reason (in over 75% of cases) for requesting reversal was the wish to share parenthood with a new partner (Lambert et al., 1984). Of this large group of requests, only a small fraction concerned women whose marriage had been ended by the death of their husband or who were already divorced or single before sterilization. The majority had divorced after their sterilization. Marital discord had been the immediate reason for sterilization of a considerable proportion of these women. In cases where the husband had made the decision or had forced his wife to be sterilized by threatening to leave her, the marriage had usually been dissolved (Poma, 1980; and Leader et al., 1983), often within months after the sterilization (Winston, 1977). Poma (1980) reported that 39% of the new partners were younger than the women. Only 12% of the new partners were more than 40 years old. Many of the younger men had not been married before, and a high proportion were childless. Murray (1980) reported that 25% of the women with new partners 'felt it necessary for a successful reversal to occur prior to remarriage and commonly stated that their new partner would not agree to marriage until the patient became pregnant'.

Requests for reversal from women who have remained in relationships

Death of a child

This was the second most common reason for reversal. Most of the cases were cot deaths which occurred between the day of sterilization and some months after the child's birth. Almost all the mothers had undergone post-partum sterilization. A smaller group of women had lost their child or children in a traffic accident or fire. The reasons stated for reversal requests varied. Some of the women (or couples) wanted to restore what Domoch (1981) called 'the family-dream'. In the case of small families, the loneliness of a remaining child for whom a brother or sister should be provided was often mentioned as a motive. A considerable proportion of the women applied for reversal within weeks or months after the tragedy, stating that they had regretted sterilization the moment the child had died (Lambers et al., 1982; and Leader et al., 1983). Lambers et al. (1982) stated they were still in deep mourning and the request for reversal seemed to be a way of coping with their grief. Others came one to three years after the event, when they had more or less worked through their grief.

Wish for more children

A considerable proportion of the women who came with the same partner (8%) gave the wish to have more children as the main reason for the request. There were several reasons at the basis of this wish. These included changed circumstances of life, such as better social and financial conditions, improved marital relationships, husbands more mature, children having grown up and left home (Thomson and Templeton, 1978; Poma, 1980; Lambers et al., 1982). Others had decided to seek reversal because of changes in medical science. For women sterilized on a medical indication the availability of amniocentesis had led some to consider pregnancy again (Winston, 1977; Thomson and Templeton, 1978).

Poma (1980) reported that 5% of his series had expected that their tubes would become 'untied' by themselves, and when nothing happended they decided to seek medical help. Another 4% had acquired new religious beliefs that regarded sterilization as interference with God's will.

Negative effects attributed to sterilization

Various negative effects of a psychological or somatic nature attributed to sterilization were mentioned as the major reason for requesting a reversal by a relatively small group of women (about 4%). This group predominantly comprised women who felt defeminized and incomplete and whose sexuality had deteriorated after the sterilization (Winston, 1977; Thomson and Templeton, 1978; Lambers *et al.*, 1982). These women could not accept the loss of their reproductive capacity, because it had been the most important part of their female identity. Many of them suffered from depression and psychosomatic complaints (Lambers *et al.*, 1982). Often these women had been sterilized for medical indications or in conjunction with an obstetric or gynecological event. Negative effects of sterilization were mentioned as secondary reasons by many women.

Religious feelings of guilt were found mostly in Catholic women (Winston, 1977). The somatic complaints of pelvic pain and menstrual troubles reported by Poma (1980) and Winston (1977) could in some cases have been psychosomatic displacement of regret (Stock, 1978), but this was not discussed by these authors.

To summarize, the incidence of regret leading to reversal request is small — approximately 5% — and seems to be greater if the sterilization was performed on a medical indication, if the sterilization was related to a recent pregnancy (particularly an abortion), if marital problems existed at the time of sterilization, and if the woman was less than 35 years old at the time of sterilization.

It might be concluded that in order to lower the incidence of reversal-request stricter criteria should be applied before performing sterilization. As 95% of sterilized women appear to be satisfied with the decision, Lambers *et al.* (1984) concluded that this would seem unrealistic and unreasonable and may lead to a very satisfactory form of definitive contraception being withheld from a substantial group of women. The best prevention of 'regret' lies in an adequate assessment and counselling of the couple.

CLINICAL IMPLICATIONS

Whilst being inconclusive, the literature provides sufficient indication to the clinician that the decision to choose tubal ligation as the means of fertility control should only be taken by patients who are well informed as to its effects and outcome. The decision should be an informed one of the couple after both have been adequately counselled about contraceptive alternatives; it should not be taken in haste or under the pressure of external factors. Special care should be taken with those patients who may be more vulnerable to the stress of tubal sterilization.

Factors associated with vulnerability

Although there is some disagreement, certain themes emerge from the literature which indicate to the clinician those women who may be at risk for adverse sequelae and who, therefore, need more careful counselling before they reach a final decision about terminating their fertility.

Age

It has been suggested that young women are at more risk for an adverse reaction to tubal ligation (Sim et al., 1973; Winston, 1977); however, there are contradictory findings (Cooper et al., 1982).

Marital problems

Several studies indicate that patients who experienced adverse sequelae following sterilization, expressed regret or requested reversal had also been experiencing marital disharmony at the time of the decision to have sterilization. Several authors recommend that patients who are experiencing marital problems at the time of their request for sterilization should receive counselling in relation to the marital problem, as concerns about fertility are likely to be only one aspect of the factors involved in such relationships. In these cases, changing circumstances such as separation, reconciliation, or a new marriage may alter the patient's view of sterilization. It is interesting to note that the majority of patients in Winston's (1977) study asking for reversal had new partners at the time of their request.

Parity

Early studies frequently cited low parity as a risk factor. However, recent studies do not support this (Smith, 1979; Cooper *et al.*, 1982), perhaps reflecting changing community attitudes to family size. In a follow-up of forty-five nulliparous women who had undergone tubal ligation, Benjamin *et al.* (1980) found that 11.4% of the women expressed unhappiness about their operation; but for most of these women the surgery was performed for medical reasons.

Previous psychiatric history and personality factors

Some studies report an association between pre-operative psychiatric history and adverse outcome. Others do not. Personality variables were found to be associated with outcome in other studies. The conclusion of Emens and Olive (1978) was that previous psychiatric illness should not be a contra-indication for sterilization but that women with severe personality disorders are likely to be dissatisfied.

Timing of surgery

The consensus of studies is clearly that there are less undesirable sequelae when women undergo interval and elective sterilization than when the operation is performed immediately after the last pregnancy.

Post-partum sterilization or sterilization combined with a therapeutic abortion or Caesarean section are found to be especially hazardous in this respect. Both occur when the woman is already in hospital or will be anesthetized, but both delivery and therapeutic abortion are highly emotional events for women. Under the pressure of these situations, a rational, well-considered decision is not always to be expected. Moreover, a woman who must have a therapeutic abortion may sometimes punish herself for allowing it by relinquishing her fertility, or she may confuse regret about the abortion with her feelings about sterilization. The practice maintained in some institutions of providing therapeutic abortion on condition of sterilization will unquestionably lead to dissatisfied, unhappy women, and should be ended (Leader *et al.*, 1983).

Pathways to surgery

This area has received little attention but some authors note that those patients who requested sterilization themselves had better outcomes than those patients who had been 'persuaded' or to whom this course had been 'suggested'. Elective sterilization solely to prevent pregnancy because no more or no children are wanted is associated with the most positive reactions (Rubenstein et al., 1979), whereas medical, psychiatric and social indications are reported by most authors to be associated with higher percentages of regret.

Counselling for reversal

For both sterilization and reversal, it must be established whether the operation is the right solution for a woman's or the couple's problem and whether the request is equally supported by both partners. Complete information must be given to the couple on the chance of operability, the chance of pregnancy after the reversal operation, and the chance of ectopic pregnancy and its consequences. All this must be discussed with the patients, and also whether they will be able to bear the strain of an uncertain period after the operation, when month after month they might try in vain to conceive, waiting before every menstrual period for possible signs of pregnancy. When confronted with the limitations and risks of a reversal operation, many patients will state that they wish to have 'done everything possible' and that under this condition they will be able to cope with a disappointment. For patients who have a new relationship it will be necessary to estimate and discuss the stability of the relationship and whether the wish for children is felt by both partners.

When a request for reversal is made because of the loss of a child, it should be established whether the mourning for the deceased child has been worked through sufficiently. Counselling might therefore be used to help parents with the mourning process. This may sometimes result in a withdrawal of the request, when after resolving grief the parents no longer feel the necessity for another child. Lambers et al. (1984) advise laparoscopy to show whether reversal of the sterilization is possible. If operation proved possible, it could be delayed, but the knowledge that refertilization might eventually be attained would also make it easier for the couple to delay the operation and first work on resolving grief.

When there is a wish for more children in the same relationship, counselling should be used to find out whether the goals of these patients might not be reached better by other means. If psychological problems or somatic complaints are given as reasons for a reversal request, the etiology of the complaints needs careful assessment.

REFERENCES

Alder, E. (1984). Sterilization. In Browne, A. and Wallace, L., (eds) *Psychology and Gynaecological Problems*, pp i–17. Tavistock, London

Alder, E., Cook, A., Gray, J., Tyrer, G., Warner, P. and Bancroft, J. (1981). The effects of sterilization: a comparison of sterilized women with the wives of vasectomised men. *Contraception*, **23**, 45–54

Ansari, J. M. A. and Francis, H. H. (1976). A study of 49 sterilized females. *Acta Psychiat. Scand.*, **54**, 315–22

Benjamin, L, Rubenstein, L. M. and Kleinkopf, V. (1980). Elective sterilization in childless women. *Fertil. Steril.*, **34**, No. 2

Cliquet, R. L., Thiery, M., Staelens, R. and Lambert, G. (1981). Voluntary sterilization in Flanders. *J. Biosoc. Sci.*, **13**, 47–61

Cooper, P. (1983). Risk of hysterectomy after sterilization. *Lancet*, **1**, 59

Cooper, C., Gath, D., Rose, N. and Fieldsend, R. (1982). Psychological sequelae to elective sterilization in women: a prospective study. *Br. Med. J.*, **284**, 461–4

Domoch, W. (1981). Regretted sterilization — Psychodynamic aspects of refertilization. In Nijs, P. and Brosens, I. (eds) *Reversibility of Sterilization, Psycho(patho)logical Aspects*. Acco, Leuven

Emens, M. J. and Olive, J. E. (1978). Timing of female sterilization. *Br. Med. J.*, **2**, 1126

Enoch, D. M. and Jones, K. (1975). Sterilization: A review of 98 sterilized women. *Br. J. Psychiat.*, **127**, 583–7

Jackson, P. (1980). Female sterilization: a five year follow-up in Auckland. *NZ Med. J.*, **91**, 140–3

Kasonde, J. M. and Bonnar, J. (1976). Effect of sterilization on menstrual blood loss. *Br. J. Obstet. Gynaecol.*, **83**, 572–5

Lambers, K. J., Trimbos-Kemper, T. and van Hall, E. V. (1982). Motivation for sterilization and subsequent wish for reversal in 70 women. *J. Psychosomat. Obstet. Gynaecol.*, **1**, (1), 17–21

Lambers, K. J., Trimbos-Kemper, T. and van Hall, E. V. (1984). Regrets and reversal of sterilization. In Broome, A. and Wallace, L. (eds) *Psychology and Gynaecological Problems*. Tavistock, London

Leader, A. Galan, N., George, R. and Taylor, P. J. (1983). A comparison of the definable traits in women requesting reversal of sterilization and women satisfied with sterilization. *Am. J. Obstet. Gynecol.*, **145**, (2), 198–202

Murray, J. (1980). A review of women requesting reversal of tubal sterilization. *Aust. NZ J. Obstet. Gynaecol.*, **20**, (4), 211–13

Neil, J. R., Hammond, G. T., Noble, A. D., Rushton, L. and Letchworth, A. T.(1975). Late complications of sterilization by laparoscopy and tubal ligation — a controlled study. *Lancet*, **2**, 699–700

Poma, P. A. (1980). Why women seek reversal of sterilization. *J. Natl. Med. Assoc.*, **71**, (1), 41–8

Rubenstein, L. M., Benjamin, L. and Kleinkopf, V. (1979). Menstrual patterns and women's attitudes following sterilization by Falope ring. *Fertil. Steril.*, **31**, (6), 641–6

Schwyhart, W. R. and Kutner, S. J. (1973). A reanalysis of female objections to contraceptive sterilization. *J. Nerv. Ment. Dis.*, **156**, 354–70

Sim, M., Emens, J. M. and Jordan, J. A. (1973). Psychiatric aspects of female sterilization. *Br. Med. J.*, **3**, 222–330

Smith, W. H. (1979). Psychiatric aspects of sterilization: a prospective survey. *Br. J. Psychiat.*, **135**, 304–9

Stock, R. J. (1978). Evaluation of sequelae of tubal ligation. *Fertil. Steril.*, **29**, (2), 169–74

Templeton, A. A. and Cole, S. (1982). Hysterectomy following sterilization. *Br. J. Obstet. Gynaecol.*, **89**, 845–8

Thomson, P. and Templeton, A. (1978). Characteristics of patients requesting reversal of sterilization. *Br. J. Obstet. Gynaecol.*, **85**, (3), 161–4

Winston, R. M. L. (1977). Why 103 women asked for reversal of sterilization. *Br. Med. J.*, **2**, 305–7

Chapter 10

The Menopause

INTRODUCTION

Scientifically, the menopause may be defined as the moment of the last uterine bleeding governed by ovarian hormonal functioning. Endocrinologically, the menopause represents the broader concept of progressive ovarian functional failure. For most women this coincides with what is commonly understood to be the years of middle-age (40–60). Endocrinological changes hence occur during a phase of life associated with psycho-social stress. Psychological and sexual complaints are frequent amongst menopausal patients. The association between these complaints and the menopause has been one of the most contentious issues in menopause research. The diversity of opinions has often reflected the discipline of the investigator. Gynecologists initially declared all such symptoms to be the 'ills' arising from an estrogen-deficiency state. Later, only vasomotor symptoms and vaginal atrophy were allowed as 'true' symptoms of the menopause. Social scientists have maintained the viewpoint that psychological and sexual complaints occurring in mid-life are not causally related to underlying biological changes but rather reflect expectations and attitudes of the particular socio-cultural group. More recently a common meeting ground for disciplines seems to have been found, with recognition of the interactive effects of endocrine changes with socio-cultural and psychological factors in any individual.

This chapter considers the relative roles of biological, psychological and sociological factors in the etiology and management of behavioural complaints.

PSYCHOLOGICAL SYMPTOMATOLOGY

Psychological symptoms of the menopause are reported to include diminished energy and drive, difficulty with concentration, irritability, aggressiveness, nervous exhaustion, fluctuations in mood, tension, depression, introversion, sense of internal frustration and inadequacy, intolerance of loneliness, marital troubles, and antisocial behaviour patterns, as well as anxiety, headache and insomnia. These symptoms are multiplicative, ill-defined and non-specific. All may occur at any age and in either sex. Such symptoms also occur in certain major psychiatric disorders, especially those of generalized anxiety and depression, and these disorders must be considered as differential diagnoses. In most cases the symptoms presented are less severe than those of anxiety and depressive neuroses, and not continuous but fluctuating.

Population studies have attempted to examine the relationship of psychological symptoms to chronological age and menopausal status. Many of these studies were reviewed previously (Dennerstein and Burrows, 1978). A number of studies reported evidence which suggested that many minor psychological changes (such as nervousness, irritability, headaches, depression and decreased social adaptation) occur in greater frequency in women whose menstrual cycles have changed recently. In a study of 800 38–60-year-old women in Gothenburg Hällström (1973) found a significant deterioration in mental health in women with irregular menstruation who were in the immediate pre-menopause.

These results were confirmed in a more recent study. Bungay et al. (1980) studied by postal questionnaire a representative sample of the Oxford population. Menopausal status was not assessed, the authors assuming a mean age of menopause of 50 years with a standard deviation of three years. A peak incidence of hot flushes and night sweats occurred with the mean age of menopause. Rising in the fifth decade and peaking in the years just prior to 50 were such symptomatology as loss of confidence, difficulty in making decisions, anxiety, forgetfulness, difficulty in concentration, feelings of unworthiness, tiredness, dizzy spells and palpitations. A different pattern was observed for the symptoms of irritability, low backache and aching breasts. These symptoms had a high prevalence throughout the years 30–50 and then began to decline.

Winokur (1973) examined the relationship between menopausal status and affective disorder requiring psychiatric admission. He found that menopausal status did not produce an increased risk of hospitalization for affective disorder over that expected for age. The peak incidence of depressive states is in the years 30–40.

SEXUAL COMPLAINTS

Loss of interest in sex and decreased responsiveness are frequent complaints of women attending menopause clinics. 70% of women attending a Sydney menopause clinic reported sexual problems. Sexual dysfunctions were often present in both partners, with many males relating onset or aggravation of their difficulties to their partner's menopause.

Epidemiological studies have sought to demonstrate whether a sudden change in sexuality occurs at the menopause, or whether there was a steady change with increasing age.

Pfeiffer *et al.* (1972) showed a dramatic decline in the sexual interest of women between the years 45 and 55. A parallel decline in male sexual interest was not evident. Hällström (1977) also found dramatic declines in the sexual interest, capacity for orgasm and coital frequency of women in the middle years of life. A fundamental question was whether the observed decrease in sexuality was related to a progressive decline due to chronological ageing or to the menopause. Hällström was able to demonstrate that decreased sexual functioning was significantly associated with menopausal status rather than with age. While recognizing that considerable individual variations existed, he noted that the majority of the post-menopausal women reported impairment of their sexual interest during the previous five years. Further confirmatory evidence was provided by the first longitudinal study of women through the climacteric years (McCoy *et al.*, 1985). In this study sixteen women kept daily calendars of intercourse occurrence and were interviewed every four months. There was a marked decline from pre- to post-menopause in sexual interest, frequency and responsiveness and this coincided with the onset of menstrual cycle irregularity. Morrell *et al.* (1984) demonstrated in a psychophysiological study that post-menopausal women (who were not receiving hormones) were significantly less responsive to erotic films, as measured by vaginal pulse amplitude, than were either young regularly menstruating women or older premenopausal women.

Hence both psychological and sexual changes begin prior to actual menopause, during a phase of altered ovarian function.

ETIOLOGY

This section considers the relative roles of biological, psychological and social factors in the behavioural changes described.

Biological

This viewpoint ascribes symptomatology to declining ovarian function. Psychological complaints may reflect a change in brain, and in particular hypothalamic, function with changing levels of steroids. The endocrine change responsible for the symptoms may be lowered levels of estrogens, progesterone or both, or raised levels of follicle stimulating hormone (FSH) and luteinizing hormone (LH). Alternatively, symptoms could reflect an imbalance elsewhere in the hypothalamic pituitary-gonadal axis. Evidence is accumulating that amine metabolism might be affected by levels of endogenous and exogenous steroid hormones. Altered amine metabolism might be responsible for affective disorders.

Mood changes and sexual disinterest are sometimes claimed to be secondary manifestations of disabling vasomotor symptoms such as hot flushes and sweating. That is, if the flushes cause the woman to stay awake and night-sweats necessitate her to change the bed-linen, she will report insomnia and fatigue which may lead to irritability and nervousness.

The finding of an association between increased psychological and sexual complaints and the years of changed ovarian activity could be interpreted as indicating possible causative links. Evidence of the specific effects of steroid hormones on mood and sexual response derives largely from clinical trials. There have been considerable methodological difficulties experienced in such studies.

In clinical trials there is a necessity for: adequate description of menopausal status, with evidence derived from hormone assays; adequate number in sample; valid measurements of variables and such measures to be sensitive to change; sufficient length of therapy; cross-over design to allow for interpatient variability in response and assessment of change; and reduction of bias by double-blind techniques. As women with perimenopausal complaints have been shown to be highly placebo-responsive, only those studies which were double-blind will be discussed here.

A review of six earlier double-blind studies (Dennerstein and Burrows, 1978) found that all except one reported that, compared with placebo, there was a decrease in psychological complaints such as irritability, fatigue, insomnia, anxiety and depression when estrogen was given alone or in combination with a progestin.

Fedor-Freybergh (1977) found a significant beneficial effect of estrogen on libido, sexual activity, satisfaction, experience of pleasure, sexual fantasies and capacity for orgasm.

The two largest double-blind, placebo-controlled, cross-over studies published both report improvements with estrogen therapy over placebo for a variety of psychological and sexual symptoms. Campbell and Whitehead (1977) compared two months' therapy of 1.25 mg conjugated estrogens (daily) with placebo in a short-term cross-over involving sixty-four patients with severe symptoms. Estrogen was found to be significantly more effective than placebo in alleviating twelve symptoms (hot flushes, insomnia, vaginal dryness*, irritability, poor memory*, anxiety*, worry about age*, headaches, worry about self*, urinary frequency, optimism, good spirits) and produced increased coital satisfaction. There was no change in masturbation, orgasmic or coital frequencies. In order to determine whether this improvement reflected relief of hot flushes, an analysis was made of the twenty patients who had not reported them. The asterisked variables above continued to be significantly improved by estrogens, indicating a direct positive effect of estrogen on mental status.

In the other large double-blind placebo-controlled cross-over study, Dennerstein *et al.* (1979, 1980) found significant beneficial effects on mood and sexual functioning. This study differed from earlier studies in the following ways. Firstly, all forty-nine women were of a definable endocrine status in that they had all received hysterectomy with bilateral oophorectomy for benign diseases. Secondly, there was a detailed study of mental status and sexual behaviour of the women prior to admission to the study. Women with diagnosable psychiatric disorder or with significant interpersonal conflict were excluded, as it was thought that such problems might overwhelm any hormonal influence. Only women with stable heterosexually active relationships were included, as one of the aims of the study was to measure the effects of hormones on sexual functioning. Thirdly, this study set out to separately measure the effects of an estrogen and a progestin and to compare these with placebo. The study used a cross-over design so that each woman received three months each of the following medications, the order of which was randomly allocated: ethinyl estradiol 50 µg/day; levonorgestrel 250 µg/day; 'Nordiol' — the combination of these two compounds; and placebo. Drug-taking was continuous, there being no drug-free periods between medication. If women were unable to tolerate the side-effects in any drug phase they were changed to the next drug in the sequence. Ethinyl estradiol given alone was found to have the most beneficial effect on psychological status as measured by Hamilton scores, and ordinal ratings of general well-being, depression, fatigue, anxiety, irritability and insomnia. The combination 'Nordiol' was next in beneficial effect, with norgestrel scoring slightly better than placebo. Although at least some of the effects on mood reflected alleviation of hot flushes, a significant effect of the hormones on the Hamilton Depression scores remained, suggesting a direct beneficial psychotropic effect of estrogen.

This study also found that ethinyl estradiol had a beneficial effect on female sexual desire, enjoyment, vaginal lubrication and orgasmic frequency (recorded daily) (Dennerstein *et al.*, 1980). There was a trend to norgestrel being more inhibitory. The combination pill was less beneficial than estrogen alone. Finally, when the relationship between headaches and the administration of hormones was examined, it was found that an increase in headaches occurred when therapy was changed from estrogen-containing compounds to the non-estrogens (norgestrel or placebo) (Dennerstein *et al.*, 1978a).

In a later double-blind cross-over study, Paterson (1982) studied twenty-three post-menopausal hysterectomized women. The women received three months each of either graded sequential mestranol and norethisterone or placebo. Active therapy resulted in a significant reduction in hot flushes and night-sweats and a slight improvement in insomnia, lack of energy and confidence, but no alteration in depression, anxiety, memory, tension, libido, or vaginal dryness. These findings in part confirm those of the previous studies (Dennerstein *et al.*, 1979, 1980) that when a progestin was added to estrogen beneficial effects on mood and sexual functioning were reduced.

There have been few double-blind studies on the role of androgens as part of hormone replacement therapy. Uncontrolled studies suggest significant sexual improvement in patients complaining of loss of libido who received a combined hormone implant of estradiol 50 mg and testosterone 100 mg.

Dow and Hart (1983) studied forty post-menopausal women referred for hormone replacement therapy, all of whom had reported a significant concern about a decline in sexual interest. These women were randomly allocated to one of two hormone implant treatment groups: either estradiol 50 mg alone or estradiol 50 mg and testosterone 100 mg. Comparison between the two groups revealed no significant differences on any measure. Both treatments were associated with a significant reduction in the severity of psychological, somatic and vasomotor symptoms and with a significant improvement in sexual interest, responsiveness, satisfaction, orgasmic capacity and dyspareunia. These results indicated no advantages of testosterone administration over estradiol alone for sexually unresponsive post-menopausal women. The only variable which was not improved by the hormone treatment was marital dissatisfaction. This study did not include a placebo control group and the sample was mixed endocrinologically in that some women had undergone hysterectomy and bilateral oophorectomy.

A recent study by Sherwin *et al.* (1985) attempted to overcome these flaws. These researchers studied women who had been hysterectomized and bilaterally oophorectomized for benign causes. Using a double-blind cross-over design, they injected intramuscularly, monthly for three months, two of the following substances: estrogen, testosterone, combined estrogen-testosterone, or placebo. There was a control group of ten women who were hysterectomized but not oophorectomized. Both mood and sexual functioning were measured. The oophorectomized women who received any of the hormonal preparations were significantly less depressed than the placebo group. The women treated with androgens alone had significantly higher hostility scores than all other groups. Exogenous androgen significantly enhanced the intensity of sexual desire and arousal and the frequency of sexual fantasies in the oophorectomized women. There was no effect on coital frequency. These findings suggest that the major impact of androgen in women is on sexual motivation rather than sexual activity *per se*.

To summarize, most double-blind studies have found beneficial effects of estrogens on psychological and sexual functioning. The addition of a progestin leads to less favourable results. When the effects of addition of an androgen were studied, no additional benefits on mood were found and there were observed effects on sexual interest.

Psychological

Earlier writers, of psychoanalytic background, portrayed negative viewpoints of the menopause. Freud suggested that the physical changes resulted in an increase in 'libido' beyond the level to which the 'ego' was capable of controlling instinctual drives. A 'neurosis' was then generated. An important theory is that of *loss*. Perceived losses occurring at the menopause include the depletion and decline in sexual attractiveness and usefulness and the loss of reproductive capacity. These may result in feelings of helplessness, hopelessness, disappointment and mortification. When the loss is invested with the loser's self-esteem, depression results. The women most affected by menopausal changes would be expected to be those with most investment in childbearing and childraising.

Declining sexual interest may occur secondarily to depressed mood. Hällström (1977) found a significant association of declining sexual interest with the Hamilton Rating Score for Depression and also with the personality trait of introversion (Eysenck Personality Inventory).

The importance of premorbid personality has been emphasized. Benedek (1960) claimed a better outcome for women whose 'adaptive capacity has not been exhausted by previous neurotic processes'. Hällström (1977) found that women who had enjoyed sex in younger years were more likely to maintain sexual response through the menopause.

Hällström (1973) also found a number of personality traits associated with women who became ill during the climacteric. These included increased neuroticism, guilt feelings and neurotic self-assertion. Women who became mentally ill more often reported mental illness amongst parents and a strict upbringing. They were also more likely to have suffered mental illness earlier in life.

Collins *et al.* (1983), in a small Swedish study of women seeking help at a menopause clinic, explored the relationship between underlying personality variables and psychological complaints. They found vasomotor and sleep-related symptoms were not associated with any personality variable other than that of feminine interest. Psychosomatic and psychological symptoms were significantly correlated with personality variables said to relate to anxiety-proneness. Psychological symptoms were also correlated with an external locus of control or the feeling that external factors determined one's life.

Whilst more studies are needed, important aspects for the clinician are that underlying personality factors may play a role in an individual's response to hormonal changes.

Sociological

Cross-cultural

The hypothesis of such studies is that the norms and values of a particular culture determine the significance attached to concepts such as youth, menstruation, fertility, sexuality, sterility, menopause, and ageing. Thus, more menopausal complaints are expected by women living in cultures (such as those of Western nations) which are youth-orientated, where fertility is valued and ageing punished.

Flint (1979) reported on her studies of 483 Rajput caste women in India. These women were well-nourished and large landowners.

Interview found that they reported few symptoms other than that of menstrual cycle change and eagerly awaited the menopause. Lack of symptomatology was interpreted as due to the positive changes in the woman's life following menopause. Prior to menopause these women either lived in purdah (veiled and secluded) or were not allowed the company of men. After menopause Rajput women were released from purdah and were allowed to talk and in some areas to drink with men. Older people in this culture were revered as models of wisdom and experience, so that ageing itself was not feared as a sign of impending senility.

Similar findings were reported when Arabian women were compared with women from Persia and Africa. The Arabian women reported little or no menopausal symptomatology. In their culture menopause was not viewed negatively and not seen as a crisis.

Davis (1982) studied thirty-eight women, aged 35–65, in a Newfoundland fishing village. Although these women maintained high status through mid-life, the majority reported hot flushes, tension-headaches, anxiety and tiredness in association with the menopause. Davis concluded that the biological changes of the peri-menopause may elicit a common negative response cross-culturally, regardless of women's status. This study was unique in exploring the cognitions of the women concerned and seeking to understand how they conceptualized the changes experienced. A folk explanation for the changes provided a female support system for those who experienced difficulty.

There are obviously many problems in such cross-cultural research. These include possible bias introduced by investigators, language problems and the possibility that some cultures express emotional changes in masked ways. No studies appear to have compared women from different cultures on endocrine parameters, presuming the duration and severity of endocrine changes are similar in different cultures. This may not be the case. Nevertheless, there is some evidence to suggest that cultural factors may be important in determining an individual's response to biological changes and the expression of perceived changes.

Changing roles

Some authors have argued for the 'empty nest' as the major psychosocial transition of this period of life. Recent studies have failed to find evidence to support the view that the 'empty nest' period was a time of crisis. To the contrary, Glen (1975) found that women whose children had left home were generally more satisfied than women whose children remained.

Socio-demographic variables

Factors such as employment status, social class, marital status and social network have been the subject of a number of studies with interesting and at times disparate findings. McKinlay and Jefferys (1974) failed to find any associations between symptoms and employment status, age at leaving school, social class, domestic workload, marital status and parity. Van Keep and Kellerhals (1974) studied Swiss women according to menopausal status and found that women in lower social classes had higher symptom scores, with the exception of women in the perimenopausal group, where women in the highest social class had the highest score. A study of Belgian women found that during the climacteric the effect of work was socially differentiated. For the upper socio-economic group, work outside the home is almost always favourable. This was not found for women of the lower socio-economic group. Van Keep (1983) also reported that women who were well-integrated in their environment and surrounded by friends reported fewer climacteric symptoms than those who were lonely.

Holt and Mikkelsen (quoted by Haspels and Musaph, 1981) reported that women in their Norwegian study who had a good social network tended not to suffer climacteric problems of a psychological nature. The presence of a personal income, rather than socio-economic status, was associated with less vasomotor complaints.

Life events

Many of the elements of the psycho-social transition can be described as stressful life events. These include exit events, such as death of husband, close relative or friend, or departure of children from the home, as well as entrance events such as becoming a grandparent. Hällström (1973) found a significant relationship between mental illness during the year preceding the examination and marriage disruption, serious problems with children, unhappiness at work and a large number of psycho-social stress factors. Among social variables which did not show any significant relation of this kind were social group, family income, civil state, amount of employment, childlessness and the last child having left home.

Cooke (1984) investigated the relationships between climacteric complaints, psycho-social vulnerability factors and life events. He found an increase in such events during the climacteric years. He also found that non-exit stress was associated with psychological complaints (such as depression, crying spells, panic attacks and worrying), whereas exit stress was not. Both exit and non-exit stress were required to produce elevation in 'somatic' symptomatology (faintness and dizziness, headaches and tingling or numbness in the body). Using a hierarchical regression analysis, Cooke found that loss of one's mother before the age of 11 and employment status act as vulnerability factors for life-event stress, influencing the occurrence of psychological complaints. The degree of involvement with children was directly associated with the occurrence of psychological complaints. The number of confidants available to the patient was directly associated with psychological symptomatology and had a synergistic effect with life-event stress. Thus the availability of confidants may help to diffuse life stress. Neither the level of confiding in the spouse, the number of children at home, or the quality of communication with children had any effect. Similar results were found for the 'somatic' complaints, except that the degree of involvement with the children no longer had any effect.

Interactive

These findings support an interactive bio-psycho-social model of the psychological complaints experienced in the climacteric years and have important implications for management. Underlying endocrinological changes may in themselves be sufficient to trigger emotional changes leading to distress. In other women these changes may lead to psychological complaints only when other factors are present. Such vulnerability factors include low socio-economic class, especially when combined with work outside the home, lack of a supportive social network, undesirable life events, degree of involvement with children, loss of mother before the age of 11, previous history of depression or treatment by a psychiatrist. Personality factors of anxiety-proneness have also been found to be associated with more psychological complaints.

MANAGEMENT

The first major step for the clinician is to establish the diagnosis of the symptoms presented. With regard to psychological and sexual complaints, the doctor needs full details of the presenting symptoms, their duration and association with the onset of the climacteric. He should also ask the patient whether she has any other menopausal complaints. In the history-taking, symptoms suggesting other major disorders should be sought. These include major psychiatric disorders, especially depression and generalized anxiety disorder, marital problems and/or sexual dysfunction, and mid-life crisis. A personal developmental history will give some idea of coping styles, personality and vulnerability. Details of the woman's current environment, and aspects of stress and support within this framework should be examined. Her attitudes and expectations of the menopause are also important. Information on factors which may affect response to hormones, such as responses to the oral contraceptive pill, post-partum depression or premenstrual tension, should be sought. Physical disorders (such as hypertension or diabetes) which may limit the use of hormones must be determined.

Investigations

In the post-menopausal woman, plasma follicle stimulating hormone and estradiol levels will help to determine the degree of estrogen deficiency. This may be especially useful for the climacteric woman who has psychological or sexual complaints but no vasomotor symptoms.

Therapy

An integrated approach to management is needed, aimed at reducing contributory hormonal, psychological and social stress and promoting a positive adaptation to this life phase. Aspects of therapy may thus include the following:

Explanation and reassurance

Such discussions should include the opportunity for the woman concerned to ventilate her feelings. As studies have shown that the woman with menopausal complaints may have fewer confiding relationships, the opportunity to discuss feelings, stress and distress is particularly needed.

Hormone therapy

The aim of such therapy should be to provide an optimal hormonal background. Estrogen treatment in the estrogen-deficient woman is likely to improve psychological and sexual functioning. A progestin must be added for those women with an intact uterus. The lowest dosage needed to reverse endometrial changes is recommended because of possible adverse psychological and sexual effects. These may be less if natural progesterone or progestins chemically similar to this are utilized. One month of therapy may be necessary before the patient detects any change. Testosterone may provide some additional benefit for the oophorectomized woman with low sexual interest.

Psychotropic drugs

If a major psychiatric disorder, such as depression, generalized anxiety disorder or schizophrenia, is diagnosed, then appropriate therapy should be instituted. If the clinician is not used to treating these disorders, referral to a psychiatrist may be appropriate. Depression of moderate or severe intensity usually requires psychotropic medication. Psychotherapy in conjunction with pharmacotherapy helps to resolve any intra- or interpersonal factors and improves the patient's coping skills. Hormonal therapy may be needed as well if the woman is shown to be hormone-deficient.

Other therapies

Cognitive therapy strategies may be of use in helping the patient to deal with stresses in her life. These are aimed at helping her to change her personal perception of events in her life. Such techniques may also help her to improve the quality of other social support relationships in her environment. Other counselling, such as that involved in sex therapy, may be needed. Relaxation training may be helpful for the woman for whom tension is a problem.

Finally, the benefit of patient support groups should be mentioned. These can help women to redefine their experience more positively, to increase their social network and to learn from others' progress.

REFERENCES

Bungay, G. T., Vessey, M. P. and McPherson, C. K. (1980). Study of symptoms in middle life with special reference to the menopause. *Br. Med. J.*, **2**, 181–3

Campbell, S. and Whitehead, M. (1977). Oestrogen therapy and the menopausal syndrome. *Clinics in Obstet. Gynaecol.*, **4**, 31–47

Collins, A., Hanson, U. and Eneroth, P. (1983). Post-menopausal symptoms and response to hormonal replacement therapy: influence of psychological factors. *J. Psychosomat. Obstet. Gynaecol.*, **2**, 227–33

Cooke, D. J. (1984). A psychosocial study of the climacteric. In Broome, A. and Wallace, L. (eds) *Psychology and Gynaecological Problems*, pp 243–65. Tavistock Publications, London

Davis, D. L. (1982). Women's status and experience of the menopause in a Newfoundland fishing village. *Maturitas*, **4**, 207–16

Dennerstein, L. and Burrows, G. D. (1978). A review of studies of the psychological symptoms found at the menopause. *Maturitas*, **1**, 55–64

Dennerstein, L., Laby, B., Burrows, G. D. and Hyman, G. J. (1978a). Headache and sex hormone therapy. *Headache*, **18**, 146–53

Dennerstein, L., Burrows, G. D., Hyman, G. J. and Sharpe, K. (1979). Hormone therapy and affect. *Maturitas*, **1**, 247–59

Dennerstein, L., Burrows, G. D., Wood, C. and Hyman, G. J. (1980). Hormones and sexuality: effect of oestrogen and progesterone. *Obstet. Gynaecol.*, **56**, 316–22

Dow, M. G. T. and Hart, D. M. (1983). Hormonal treatments of sexual unresponsiveness in postmenopausal women: a comparative study. *Br. J. Obstet. Gynaecol.*, **90**, 361–6

Fedor-Freybergh, P. (1977). The influence of oestrogens on the well-being and mental performance in climacterical and postmenopausal women. *Acta Obstet. Gynecol. Scand.*, **Suppl.**, 64

Flint, M. P. (1979). Sociology and anthropology of the menopause. In van Keep, P. A., Serr, D. M. and Greenblatt, R. B. (eds) *Female and Male Climacteric*, pp 1–8. MTP Press Ltd., Lancaster

Glen, N. D. (1975). Psychological well-being in the post-parental stage. Some evidence from national surveys. *J. Marriage and Fam.*, **37**, 105–10

Hällström, T. (1973). *Mental Disorder and Sexuality in the Climacteric.* Scandinavian University Books, Copenhagen

Hällström, T. (1977). Sexuality in the climacteric. In Greenblatt, R. B. and Studd, J. (eds) *Clinics in Obstetrics and Gynaecology: The Menopause*, Vol. 4, pp 227–39

Haspels, A. A. and Musaph, H. (1981). Psychosexual aspects of mid-life. In van Keep, P. A., Utian, W. H. and Vermeulen, A. (eds) *The Controversial Climacteric*, pp 39–50. MTP Press Ltd., Lancaster

McCoy, N. L. and Davidson, J. M. (1985). A longitudinal study of the effects of menopause on sexuality. *Maturitas*, **7**, 203–10

McKinlay, S. M. and Jefferys, M. (1974). The menopausal syndrome. *Br. J. Prev. Soc. Med.*, **28**, 108–15

Morrell, M. J., Dixen, J. M., Carter, C. S. and Davidson, J. M. (1984). The influence of age and cycling status on sexual arousability in women. *Am. J. Obstet. Gynecol.*, **148**, 66–71

Paterson, M. E. L. (1982). A randomised, double-blind, cross-over study into the effect of sequential mestranol and norethisterone on climacteric symptoms and biochemical parameters. *Maturitas*, **4**, 83–94

Pfeiffer, E., Verwoerdt, A. and Davis, G. C. (1972). Sexual behaviour in middle life. *Am. J. Psychiat.*, **128**, 1262–7

Sherwin, B. B., Gelfard, M. M. and Brender, W. (1985). Androgen enhances sexual motivation in females: a prospective, cross-over study of sex steroid administration in the surgical menopause. *Psychosomat. Med.*, **47**, 00–00

van Keep, P. A. and Kellerhals, J. M. (1974). The impact of socio-cultural factors on symptom formation. *Psychother. Psychosomat.*, **23**, 251–63

van Keep, P. A. (1983). The menopause. Part B: Psychosomatic aspects of the menopause. In Dennerstein, L. and Burrows, G. D. (eds) *Handbook of Psychosomatic Obstetrics and Gynaecology*, pp 483–90. Elsevier Biomedical Press, Amsterdam

Winokur, G. (1973). Depression in the menopause. *Am. J. Psychiat.*, **130**, 92–3

Chapter 11

Gynecological Cancer

by Gerjanne Bos

INTRODUCTION

The diagnosis of cancer constitutes a psychological crisis for patients and their families (Capone *et al.*, 1980). Besides the distress caused by the diagnosis, many patients report increased anxiety, depression, anger and guilt. They are overcome by a sense of loss engendered by being deprived of health and faced with the possibility of death as well as the loss of self-control, self-esteem, employment and social status. Patients with cancer feel stigmatized by society; not only the disease itself but even its name has a profound impact and triggers powerful emotional reactions. The persisting myth that cancer is contagious further isolates many patients (Sontag, 1979).

Cancer occurring in an organ associated with femininity and sexuality may well give rise to different reactions than cancer affecting a less emotionally charged site, and many authors recognize the fact that gynecological cancers are unique due to the direct impact they have on the feminine and sexual identity (Dennerstein *et al.*, 1977; Derogatis, 1980; Mantell and Green, 1978; Capone *et al.*, 1980; Holland and Mastrovito, 1980; Abitbol and Davenport, 1974; Amias, 1975; Donahue and Knapp, 1977; Vincent *et al.*, 1975). Genital organs have various kinds of important functions and values: biological, psychological, relational, sexual, and aesthetic. At different levels these factors contribute to the sense of femininity. When these female body parts are affected by malignancies, this may mean that cherished body parts are affected, security in feminine and sexual roles is assaulted, and relationships to intimate and important others are threatened (Krant, 1981). Although gynecological oncology deals with a variety of sites and degrees of danger and disfigurement, the fundamental effects on the patient's self-image are the same. The degree may vary for each individual, depending on factors such as personal history, gender role definition, and age. Thus, women — whose self-image is strongly bound to physical attributes — may have more problems in coping with the physical consequences of cancer treatment (Mastrovito, 1974). According to La Torre (1978), the same applies for extremely 'feminine' women.

Age is another factor that is related to coping with cancer. Obviously, the passage of time itself does not have a moderating effect, but the events taking place in that time do. Derogatis (1980) comments that younger women are more apt to be devastated by a cancer that may rob them of their capacity to reproduce and/or render them less desirable as a sexual or marital partner. Weideger, in her book *Menstruation and Menopause* (1976), remarks that young women fear the menopause because being menopausal is associated with being old. Surgical menopause may therefore add to the heavy burden of genital cancer. These findings are in agreement with the results of Sewell and Edwards (1980) that older women in stable relationships of considerable duration tend to have fewer problems than younger patients in shorter relationships.

In sum, the effects of gynecological cancer will differ according to site, stage, treatment, age, etc., and it is evident that many different factors will influence the way in which patients cope with their disease as well as the quality of their life afterward.

EFFECTS OF GYNECOLOGICAL CANCERS

Table 8 presents a model of the effects of gynecological cancer that covers physical, psychological and socio-cultural effects pertaining to female organs and functions, female identity and female image, which will be discussed here.

Physical effects

The incidence of gynecological cancer is second only to that of breast cancer, which in the Netherlands, unlike in some other countries, is not included among the gynecological cancers. For the Netherlands and the USA 39 and 49% of the genital malignancies originate in the endometrium, 24 and 20% in the cervix, 27 and 25% in the ovary, and 10 and 6% in the vulva and vagina, respectively (Dutch Society of Gynecologic Oncology, 1985; American Cancer Society, 1984).

Because of differences in site and stage of the disease, each site has specific physical effects in terms of loss of organs, functions and disturbances. For endometrial and cervical cancer, surgical treatment differs from simple hysterectomy (followed by radiation therapy) to a radical Wertheim's hysterectomy, which includes the removal of the upper third of the vagina, the parametria and pelvic lymphadenectomy. For ovarian cancer, surgery ranges from simple oophorectomy to total abdominal hysterectomy and bilateral salpingo-oophorectomy, including omentectomy and cytoreductive surgery in advanced cases. For vulvar cancer, surgery ranges from a simple vulvectomy for microinvasive cancer to a radical vulvectomy, including regional lymph node dissection. The inner and outer labia and entrance to the vagina are removed, and a clitoridectomy is generally necessary. For vaginal cancer and central pelvic metastases, anterior exenteration (removal of the

Table 8 Effects of gynecological cancers: a model

Physical	*Psychological*	*Socio-cultural*
Assault on female organs	*Assault on female identity*	*Assault on female image*
Ovaries, tubes, uterus, cervix, vagina, vulva, clitoris	Body image Self-esteem Integrity	Health ideal Body ideal Motherhood ideal
Loss of female functions	*Loss of 'feminine' identity*	*Loss of feminine value*
Menstruation Fertility Hormonal equilibrium	Devalued as woman Feeling incomplete, not whole	Feminine status Social status Feminine mystique
Disturbances of sexual functions	*Disturbances of sexual identity*	*Disturbances attributable to sexual norms*
Sensory perception Uterine contractions Lubrication Orgasm capacity	Devalued as sexual partner Insecure Inhibited Anorgasmic Worries about being contagious	Genital cancer seen as punishment for sexual 'sins' Sexuality is taboo for sick people Sexuality is taboo for mutilated/castrated people Non-coital sex is taboo

uterus, bladder, and part or all of the vagina), posterior exenteration (removal of the uterus, rectum, vagina) or total pelvic exenteration (removal of the bladder, uterus, rectum, vagina, pelvic floor, and perineum) may be indicated, but the incidence of these mutilating operations is nowadays very rare. Each of these operations may be combined with a vulvectomy (Perez *et al.*, 1982; Heintz and Trimbos, 1984; Trimbos, 1985). Surgery may be followed by radiotherapy and/or chemotherapy.

The physical effects of each surgery invariably cause functional losses, such as the disappearance of menstruation, loss of fertility, and hormonal disequilibrium. Moreover, these changes may in turn influence sexual functioning in ways resulting in the loss of sensory perceptions. When a Wertheim's hysterectomy is performed the vagina is considerably shortened, and the scarring may cause a decrease of vaginal elasticity. The absence of the uterus and the scar tissue replacing the cervix prevent full ballooning of the back of the vagina, and there will be no uterine contractions during orgasm. If an oophorectomy has been performed, the decreased production of estrogen may reduce the amount and rapidity of vaginal lubrication. Although the vagina itself may not have been altered, dyspareunia may result from scarring and stenosis, as is often the case in vulvar cancer. For women with vaginal or pelvic cancer, vaginal intercourse is no longer possible due to loss of the vagina. In addition, ileostomy, colostomy, or both will be necessary.

Besides the specific physical effects of gynecological cancer, general feelings of malaise may occur.

Psychological effects

Psychological effects can also differ appreciably from patient to patient and are influenced by age, personal history, phase of life, and the individual woman's characteristic coping mechanisms (Derogatis, 1980). On the psychological level, loss of female organs and functions are experienced as a violent assault on the body image and are therefore damaging to a woman's self-esteem (Holland, 1976; Vettese, 1976).

Andersen and Jochimsen (1985) compared three groups of women: patients with breast cancer, patients with gynecological cancer, and healthy women. A poor body image was reported by 82% of the gynecological cancer patients as against 38% of the healthy women and, surprisingly, 31% of the women with breast cancer.

Gynecological cancer may be experienced as a serious assault on the female identity too; a woman's positive feelings about her body are often changed into a negative body image; perceived physical unattractiveness, worthlessness and asexuality (Mantell, 1983). This disease is felt by many women, both young and old, to be unfair: 'I've always kept my body so clean', and as betrayal: 'My body has let me down'. After gynecological surgery, a woman's positive feelings about herself are also often changed into negative feelings with lowered self-esteem. Many women feel inferior and insecure: 'I'm no longer a woman'. The medical literature has linked cervical cancer with promiscuity and early sexual experience, so that the cancer may be seen by some as punishment for real or imagined sexual behaviour that may still be guilt-laden. Gynecological cancer may also have a connotation leading to feelings of shame, embarrassment, or ignorance (Bos, 1984), especially in the case of vulvar cancer. These negative feelings about body image and self-esteem may have consequences for a woman's sexual identity as well. Many women feel devalued as sexual partner, may be inhibited, because they fear to be contagious, and are concerned that they may lose their partner.

Even when gynecological surgery does not involve oncological surgery, it is abundantly clear that sexual dysfunction is attendant. In their study, Dennerstein et al. (1977) found a 37% incidence rate for sexual disorders following hysterectomy and oophorectomy even for non-malignant diseases.

Socio-cultural effects

On the socio-cultural level gynecological cancer may threaten the female image. In Western society, women are expected to be healthy, attractive and youthful, and the potential for motherhood is highly valued. The loss of female organs and functions as well as aesthetic value may be experienced as a loss of feminine value; the feminine status and mystique have suddenly disappeared and many patients perceive a diminished social status compared to that of healthy women. Traditional sexual values and norms may further add to the heavy burden for patients as well as for their partners (Bos, 1986).

It is obvious that in gynecological cancer causes are associated with and attributed to genital organs and functions. In Leiden, as part of an ongoing research project concerning the quality of life of gynecological cancer patients, fifty-three women were asked what they perceived as the cause of their disease. It is striking that about two-thirds of this group ascribed the cause to themselves and felt guilty, as against the other third, who referred to external influences. Almost half of the patients related the cause to sexuality or reproduction, whereas the others reported as causes, in descending order, stress, punishment, heredity, fate, and chance. It is evident that genital cancer can be seen as punishment and may result in avoidance of sex. Moreover, if coitus is no longer attractive or possible, couples often refrain from sex completely and, tragically, from physical intimacy as well. And although this lack of physical closeness is regretted by many women, they seem incapable of changing their traditional mutual sexual habits and patterns.

In sum, the physical, psychological and socio-cultural effects of gynecological cancer all intermingle and influence the patient's reactions to her losses as well as the way she copes with it (Schain, 1981).

PSYCHOLOGICAL IMPACT OF GYNECOLOGICAL CANCER

As an illness cancer is chronic in nature, and in optimal cases can be cured physically. The time from the first suspicious signals obtained via screening, confirmation of the diagnosis, and medical treatment to termination of the treatment by either death or cure is often quite long. In this process the following phases can be distinguished: the period around the time of diagnosis, the period of medical treatments, and — if a cure is achieved — the period of survival or remission. The terminal phase — however important — will not be discussed here. Although these periods may overlap, the psychological impact of each of them will be discussed separately.

Impact of diagnosis

For many women who have been screened for cervical cancer the diagnosis is not really unexpected, because for some time they have had complaints such as pelvic pain, coital pain, contact bleeding, or vaginal infections and the positive Papanicolaou smear was therefore anticipated. For other women, however, a positive Pap smear can be extremely confusing, especially if they have been checked regularly. Because all their previous smears were negative, they are convinced that a mistake has been made, and at first they refuse to accept this unexpected diagnosis.

For other sites of gynecological cancer this may be different. An ovarian carcinoma, for example, is present much longer before it is diagnosed and it is often discovered by chance. Affected women have often had a long period of vague but uncomfortable symptoms, and have consulted several physicians for relief of their symptoms (the so-called 'shopping pattern'). Lennane and Lennane (1973) concluded that physicians may over-emphasize psychogenic factors in dealing with female patients. If a woman displays nervous or anxious behaviour, her symptoms are more likely to be regarded as neurotic. This labelling delays early diagnosis and may also complicate adequate coping, because these women tend to blame doctors for not having taken them seriously.

Once cancer is suspected, there is a period of extensive examination and the woman alternates between the extremes of hope and despair. The uncertainty is so unbearable for some patients that they can relax — at least temporarily — only after the biopsies confirm malignancy and they know where they stand. The very moment the diagnosis is confirmed, a woman becomes a cancer patient. Patients report feeling shocked, terrified, numb, panicky or stunned.

Of the utmost importance is the way in which women are informed about their disease, and this has long-lasting effects. The majority of women are satisfied with the way in which their doctor dealt with this situation, but a minority have serious objections, for example, if they feel they have been blamed for a late diagnosis or when they have been informed while standing in a corridor or in the absence of their partner or a close relative. According to Cain *et al.* (1983), 25% of the patients in their survey had been informed by their family doctor by telephone, and these women stated unequivocally that they would have preferred being told face to face.

The information about the diagnosis must be conveyed in the right words, by the right person and under the right conditions, but the consequences of the various forms of treatment must also be presented with great care. For example, it is improper to tell a woman who is to undergo a hysterectomy that she 'luckily' already has a child.

Information about treatment may become even more important when the patient wishes to participate in decision-making about the choice and extent of therapy. According to Fox (1981): 'Almost all patients are completely unequipped to make such a choice. Even if the physician fills them in, they are usually not in any shape (partly because of their emotional state) either to apprehend the facts properly or to weigh them.' Young women find it of vital importance that the doctor discusses the effects of the treatment, especially with respect to fertility and sexuality, with them seriously and that these effects are not trivialized or left unmentioned (Bos, 1986). In general, most women seem to be quite satisfied about the medical information given to them as well as with the way in which they were informed.

Talking about the diagnosed malignancy is stressful for the patient, her family, and her physician. Many practical arrangements must be made, and many women remain absorbed in household affairs up to the day they are admitted to hospital, thus escaping from existential aspects of the disease. In case the women feel a need to talk, for instance, about the possibility of dying, they encounter little response. Many husbands ward off all thought of disaster and attempt only to reassure their wives. Real communication between husband and wife is often impossible, because they want to spare each other. This has the effect of making both feel lonely: the wife feels emotionally deserted and the husband is unable to share with her his own fears and worries. Instead, he attempts to stick to the male role pattern (because his own coping skills are inadequate); he helps her in practical matters, but emotionally he leaves her in the lurch.

The immediate reactions to the diagnosis have been studied by several investigators. Peck (1972) has reported that the most common reactions to the diagnosis of cancer are anxiety, depression, guilt, and anger. Andersen (1984) compared forty women with stage I or II gynecological cancer with forty 'healthy' women scheduled for routine gynecological examination and forty women undergoing treatment for a benign gynecological disease. The cancer group reported significantly more depression than the other two groups, and the cancer and benign groups showed comparable levels of anxiety and fatigue, whereas both symptoms occurred less frequently in the healthy group.

Cain *et al.* (1983) compared women suffering from cervical, uterine, or ovarian malignancy ($n = 60$) with a randomly selected community sample ($n = 272$) and with psychiatric female patients ($n = 40$). The cancer patients were found to be more depressive and anxious than the healthy women but had fewer symptoms than the psychiatric patients. For all sites of gynecological cancer, the level of depression and anxiety and the degree of psycho-social impairment was in the low to moderate range. Patients with cervical cancer were more anxious than patients with endometrial or ovarian cancer, but patients with ovarian cancer were more depressive than those with endometrial or cervical cancer. Comparison between stages for all tumour sites revealed no differences, whereas the histological grades were significantly differentiated: the higher the grade, the greater the psychological impairment (e.g., depression and anxiety).

From these studies it is evident that being diagnosed as having gynecological cancer causes severe distress and is accompanied by depression, anxiety, and other kinds of disturbances. The average age of the patients was very high in Cain et al.'s study (1983), moderately high in Capone et al.'s study (1980), and not indicated in Andersen's (1984) report. Thus, the effect of age on the impact of the diagnosis is unknown.

Seemingly in contradiction with the above-mentioned findings are the results of the study done by Capone et al. (1980), who compared fifty-six patients with a 'normal' population and found similar levels of emotional distress and symptoms in both groups, which the authors explained as the result of coping with the diagnosis by minimization or denial. They also agree with the findings of Vincent et al. (1975), who found that 78% of the patients with cervical cancer presented an image of being 'self-sufficient, brave, courageous, and quite able to manage their own feelings', but concluded that this image proved to be more feigned than real.

Impact of medical treatments

The diagnosis period is followed by admission to a hospital for further investigation and treatment. Hospitalization itself triggers anxiety and predisposes the patient to depression and withdrawal (Hersh, 1982). Varying amounts of depression and anxiety in patients under treatment have been reported. Some show moderately high levels and some show lower levels. Depression can be expected to be greater in those with more advanced stages of the disease on the grounds that they would anticipate earlier death or have less hope of being cured (Fox, 1981).

Many studies have shown that patients who know what to expect before treatment is started cope better than uninformed patients (Langer et al., 1975; Sime, 1976; Reading, 1981; Johnston, 1980). Research has also shown that a substantial proportion of the information given to patients is not assimilated, due to the high levels of anxiety, even in women undergoing minor gynecological surgery (Reading, 1981; Wallace, 1984).

Impact of breast surgery

Most of these patients want to have the operation as soon as possible, the sooner the better. They want to get rid of the cancer without delay, and have everything 'bad' removed. The prospect of an operation often induces anxiety, which is frequently revealed in vivid dreams and nightmares. Many patients visualize their mutilated body, their death, or their funeral (Sutherland and Orbach, 1953).

After the period of panic and restlessness at home, for most of the patients being in the hospital bed is the first time they are alone with their body and thoughts. One of our patients described lying in bed on the last night before the operation and touching the still intact smooth skin of her belly. It was the first time she cried.

Although fears about surgery can be based on more than one expectation, some of the main single sources of anxiety are mentioned in the pioneering study on the psychological impact of cancer and cancer surgery performed by Drellich, Bieber and Sutherland (1956). First, there is the fear of surgery and of the pain itself. Surgery for gynecological cancer can take many hours, and women wonder what will be cut out and how. The fear of dying during surgery is often unspoken but always there. A patient who is the mother of young children wonders how they will manage without her, and others think about whether their husband will take a second wife. Another source of stress is the fear of loss of consciousness and loss of self-control. Some women anticipate disagreeable psot-anesthesia reactions such as nausea and dizziness.

After the operation the patients are grateful to their doctor and to God because they are 'alive again'. Each day they feel better. They enjoy the many tokens of the warmth and love of family and friends, and they take pleasure in being cared for by the doctors and hospital staff. They are mainly preoccupied with their physical state; the psychological problems are set aside while they use all their energy to recover quickly so that they can go home.

Impact of radiotherapy

Radiotherapy can be used alone or in combination with surgery or chemotherapy. The most frequent side-effects of radiotherapy are fatigue, appetite loss, pain, nausea and vomiting. Late radiation treatment side-effects are vaginal atrophy and stenosis resulting in libido loss and dsypareunia. Radiotherapy may be a frightening treatment, especially when intravaginal or intrauterine radiation is performed, the intracavitary radiotherapy (ICR). In that case patients have to be nearly isolated, which may elicit claustrophobic reactions. The most frequently reported fears associated with radiotherapy are of being 'burned', becoming sterile, and developing a secondary tumour.

Little is known about the psychological impact of radiotherapy. Peck and Boland (1977) interviewed fifty patients receiving treatment for potentially curable cancer and found anxiety more frequently than any other emotional response. In their series, 60% of the patients had significant anxiety prior to treatment and 80% afterwards. Andersen *et al*. (1984) investigated women's response to ICR and found high levels of anxiety before treatment but also twenty-four hours afterwards.

Since the results of radiotherapy can be assessed only many months after the end of the treatment, many patients are left with uncertainty about its effectiveness. This can influence post-treatment anxiety and interfere with adequate coping.

Impact of chemotherapy

In this group of patients in the Netherlands, chemotherapy is mainly an adjuvant therapy for ovarian cancer. As a form of treatment, chemotherapy is extremely heavy. The repeated periods of administration of several kinds of cytostatic drugs are spread over six months to two years, which requires repeated hospitalization and produces considerable physical and psychological suffering (Small *et al*., 1983). These forms of treatment are accompanied by a wide range of side-effects, including nausea, vomiting, diarrhea, general malaise, hair loss, and loss of taste, appetite, and libido. The accompanying psychic stress is characterized by feelings of helplessness, personal failure, despair, anger and depression (Cohn, 1982; Brinkley, 1983).

Cain *et al*. (1983) investigated the psychological reactions related to chemotherapy and found that the symptoms of depression experienced by patients with ovarian cancer given triple-agent chemotherapy approached the level seen in psychiatric patients. The authors added that this finding must be understood within the context of the organic realities of the treatment. In this connection it may be mentioned that in a study on affective and cognitive effects of chemotherapy in cancer patients, Silberfarb *et al*. (1980) found that high levels of emotional distress could be attributed to disturbed physiology rather than to psychogenic causes.

The knowledge that a period of sickness and ill-health must be endured without any certainty that the treatment will be successful makes perseverance a matter of faith. Only a large reserve of courage and a fighting spirit can make it possible to complete the treatment. Interviews and psychotherapeutic interventions in patients in Leiden have shown that many of them admit to having considered giving up the battle, pulling out the plug, or throwing the pills away; suicidal thoughts are far from rare. The treatment makes such heavy demands that they say they would have been unable to complete it without the support of others, e.g., their husband and children. One patient put it into words as follows: 'I finally flushed the pills down the toilet, I could not go on, I was broken. Then the family took over and pulled me through.' It is more than clear that the treatment puts an enormous load not only on the family but also on the hospital staff, and that the support and comfort given by the medical staff and the nurses contribute in a high degree to the well-being of the patient and are gratefully remembered even years later. From the very beginning, the patients must fight to get better, which means that their attitude and share in the treatment are determinative for the effect. For some of them this implies that patients who do not recover did not try hard enough, an incorrect and dangerous conclusion that is only too common.

For patients it may be very discouraging to see the shrinking of the group of now familiar patients, reported as follows: 'You start with ten to fifteen patients and in no time at all only a couple are left. You begin to think "how soon is my turn coming?"' Even when at long last the specialist tells the patient that she has had her last course of chemotherapy she hardly dares to allow herself to think that she has become a survivor, put into words as: 'It's a miracle, I've made it!'

QUALITY OF LIFE IN SURVIVORS

Survival rates have increased significantly for cancer patients (Cullen, 1981; De Vita, 1982; Newell *et al.*, 1982; Murphy, 1984). With earlier diagnosis and combined treatments more women with gynecological cancer now survive for at least five years (Perez *et al.*, 1982; Donahue and Knapp, 1977; Ayres, 1984). It might be wondered whether the expense and pain of cancer treatment are wasted if the patient's identity and basic trust, body image, self-esteem, peace of mind, partner and sexual relationship, social roles and relations, and employment are all diminished or inferior, i.e., if the quality of life of survivors is negative. The impact of cancer and cancer treatment on the quality of life is realized by many well-known investigators, some of whom have concluded that: 'Simply staying alive may not suffice.' (Golden and Golden, 1980).

What do cancer patients do in later life, and do they still consider themselves to be 'patients' who engage in 'illness behaviour' (Cohen, 1982)?

'Because cancer is a chronic rather than an acute disease, attention must be given not only to keeping the patient alive, but also to the quality of that life' (Clark, 1976; Spinetta, 1981). Fortunately, this attention is increasing in training and research as well. For example, the problem of the quality of life had the highest priority in the postgraduate course on 'Current Concepts in Psycho-Oncology' organized by the Memorial Sloan-Kettering Cancer Center in New York (1984). From a study on the quality of life of long-term survivors treated with radiotherapy, Danoff et al. (1983) concluded that the overall impact of the disease and treatment on the patient's perceived well-being tends to be underestimated by physicians. In a similar survey performed by the American Cancer Society, physicians felt a need for discussion of problems in only 20% of their patients, whereas 80% of these cancer patients and their families felt this need (Luce, 1979). Furthermore, psychic problems are rarely apparent to the hospital staff. Patients and their relatives are reluctant to disclose their difficulties to those involved in their physical care; they give few verbal clues and perceive doctors and nurses as being primarily concerned with their physical well-being (Morris et al., 1977; Maguire et al., 1978).

In a recent handbook on the psycho-social aspects of cancer, one of the editors summarized the source of concern as follows: 'Five-year cure rates and long remissions are of little consequence if the patient's quality of life and state of wellness are less than optimal to him. In order to place the psychosocial needs of the cancer patient in perspective, there is a need for greater understanding and treatment of his emotional and social problems.' (Martin, 1982).

Short-term survival

Weisman and Worden (1976–7) found that during the first hundred days of being a cancer patient concern is predominantly existential in nature and is centred around death and life. In this early post-treatment period, worries about physical symptoms and health are dominant. Only after the patient recovers and gains some trust in the idea that she has a future and that her body seems likely to survive do psychic problems gradually become more noticeable. Often, the psychic distress does not become manifest until six to nine months after treatment (Mantell and Green, 1978; Lamont et al., 1978; Krant, 1981; Bloom and Ross, 1982). The saying that time heals all wounds certainly does not hold for coping with cancer; quite the opposite: time seems to disclose the wounds.

After the initial and relatively rapid recovery from surgery, the course of further physical recovery is much slower and therefore for most of the patients very disappointing. Patients report that in this phase they miss the protection of the hospital, feel themselves abandoned with their worries about bodily sensations and pains, and miss the attention and reassurance of the nurses and doctors. They must become reacquainted with the body which has disappointed them and which is still strange to them. Feelings of depersonalization are often reported: a young girl of 20 who had been treated for ovarian cancer said that she had become a stranger to herself and her body: 'It's not my body any longer, it feels hostile.' When the interval between diagnosis and treatment is short — e.g., only a few weeks, as is often the case for cervical cancer — many doubts may arise about the need for such radical surgery. 'Since I heard that the tissue they took out was clean, I have been wondering whether such a big operation was really necessary.' Or, 'Why couldn't I have had a baby first? What was all the rush?' Looking back to that time of panic and haste, patients wonder whether a more conservative form of treatment would have been adequate and hold their physician responsible for the organ loss. We must keep in mind that many patients with cervical cancer have only had 'cancer for a fortnight'; they 'forget' that they have had cancer and often remark that 'it is like a bad dream', and are far from being ready to cope with cancer.

There is initially a denial or avoidance of cancer, that is gradually followed by awareness, a common adjustment after traumas.

Long-term survival

Everything has its time. This also holds for what people can manage emotionally at a certain point in time. If recovery takes a turn for the better, a shift occurs from the primitive worries about existence and the body to the psyche. At first, patients have to cope with existential questions, then they have to cope with physical problems, and finally, in order to cure psychologically, they have to cope with their 'new' life.

The way in which coping occurs and the extent to which it is completed is determined by the patient's age, the degree of organ loss, the personal situation, the positive or negative social support, flexibility, etc. It is surprising that the majority of patients cope adequately, but a minority fail to do so and develop psychological or even psychiatric morbidity (Lazarus, 1982).

The prevalence of psychological morbidity is rather high, amounting to between 22 and 33% of the cancer patients (Morris *et al.*, 1977; Maguire *et al.*, 1978; Lloyd, 1979; Holland, 1976). Derogatis *et al.* (1983) assessed the prevalence of psychiatric disorders among cancer patients and found a rate of 47% for DSM-III (Diagnostic and Statistical Manual of Mental Disorders) defined psychiatric disorders. Of these cases, however, more than two-thirds concerned reactive types of adjustment disorder and the other 13% were major depressive disorders, i.e., the same distribution as for the general population.

In their investigation of psychological morbidity among one hundred cancer survivors, Mages *et al.* (1980) emphasize three distinct periods: 1) initial turmoil; 2) the period of trying different coping mechanisms; and 3) the ultimate formation of a relatively stable adaptive pattern that may be quite different from the one that prevailed before the diagnosis.

Fobair and Mages (1981), in a report of a study on psycho-social morbidity among thirty-five long-term survivors, underscore the importance of viewing the response to cancer as extending over time. Some of the patients experienced positive changes, but most had a less favourable self-image than they had had in health, and a more constricted life. These authors point to the persistence of maladaptive patterns once established.

Gottesman and Lewis (1982) studied differences in crisis reactions among cancer and surgery patients, and found not only that cancer patients feel more helpless than patients undergoing other major surgery but also that cancer patients take longer to resolve the emotional impact of the experience.

Danoff *et al.* (1983) compared the quality of life of long-term survivors and found that, compared with patients with cancer at other sites, patients with gynecological malignancies and lymphomas were significantly less satisfied with their social life and with the amount of enjoyment they had from living, which might mean that the quality of their life is lower than that of any group of survivors of cancer at other sites.

For patients with gynecological cancer at various sites, Andersen (1984) reported a significant decline in distress after four months of treatment compared to the level at diagnosis and an increase at follow-up after eight and twelve months.

Sewell and Edwards (1980) studied forty-six patients who had undergone surgery for gynecological cancer and compared effects after three types of surgery, i.e., the Wertheim's hysterectomy, radical vulvectomy, and pelvic exenteration. Six months after the operation, these authors found significant negative changes in body image, sexuality, and interpersonal relationships. The occurrence of these changes in the Wertheim's group was unexpected. However, the patients in this group were much younger (mean age: 40 years) than was the case in the other groups (mean age in both: 55 years). This suggests that age and the related life stage may be more decisive for the quality of life than site and stage of the disease.

Psychological problems become important later. For many patients this shift is rather unexpected and some think this psychic collapse is a form of 'madness', whereas others feel as though they have returned to adolescence. They feel insecure, have less self-confidence, and are not in harmony with themselves; in short, they are psychically dislocated. Frequently, their relationships with those around them are not as they would wish them to be, and this makes them feel helpless and disappointed. Many of them are reduced to despair by remarks to the effect that now they are better and can stop making a fuss. They are glad they have recovered, but that is just where the difficulty lies. The impact of the treatment and their sadness about organ losses and functions are realized to the full extent and awareness. They have just begun the process of mourning and coping. Another remark they have trouble with is: 'Now you are better you can be your old self again', but that too is impossible for the cancer patient who has been profoundly changed and can never again be as before.

Quality of life research project Leiden

In Leiden, a pilot study on the quality of life of gynecological cancer patients and their needs of and possibilities for short-term psychotherapy is nearly finished as part of a broad research project (Bos *et al.*, 1986). A broader project is funded by the Netherlands Cancer Foundation KWF for four years and will take another two years to complete. The aims of the study are: to identify patients with psychological morbidity or low quality of life; to improve the quality of life of medically-treated cancer patients; and to evaluate the results of short-term psychotherapy.

Preliminary findings can be reported from fifty-three women treated for different kinds of gynecological cancer. They were all cured, or at least nine months in remission.

It was found that age and life stage may influence the degree of psychological distress. Up to the age of 20 years hardly any distress is reported, which does not mean that problems will not become manifest later in time. Complaints are most frequent in the age group between 20 and 50 years, whereas in women over 50 years they again diminish. The interpretation could be that the psychological consequences of gynecological cancer are less serious at older ages or that they are under-reported or 'swallowed'. Another interesting finding is that three-quarters of the women in the age group of 20–30 years feel less powerful than before their disease.

The responses to questionnaires also showed that for many women the body image changed negatively: one-third considered their body to be less attractive than before the operation and two-thirds had problems with scars from the operation.

Cancer also has social consequences. One-third of the women felt more lonely than before the disease. The cancer taboo still retains its potency. More than 40% of the women concealed their experience with cancer from most people and again 40% felt ashamed at having had this disease.

From questionnaires, interviews and psychotherapy, it became evident that patients who become infertile and have a child wish, and women treated with chemotherapy are in the high-risk group for psychological morbidity (Bos, 1986; Bos, in press). It was also found that partners or husbands of cancer patients belong to a neglected group.

The results of interviews stress great differences in coping with cancer. In order to improve coping skills and coping styles, with the ultimate goal of improving the quality of life of cured patients, psychotherapy on an individual or group basis was offered to all women and accepted by many. Referral for psychotherapy should be seriously considered by physicians as being a treatment 'par excellence' to improve a diminished quality of life.

SUMMARY AND CONCLUSIONS

The subjective quality of life of a patient cured of, or in remission of gynecological cancer is determined by a diversity of effects and factors. First of all, the physical effects of the different sites, stages and treatments and the extent of resulting loss of organs and functions. Then, the psychological effects and the extent of anxiety, depression, loss of body image, self-esteem and female identity. Thirdly, the socio-cultural effects and the extent to which they influence the patient and her social context. These major effects also influence sexual functions, sexual identity and the sexual relationship more or less strongly.

Besides the effects due to cancer and cancer treatment, there are other important factors which determine a patient's quality of life after survival, such as: age, life-stage, past history, social support, sexual, female, and social role patterns, sexual preference, etc. All illness and treatment effects, together with personal factors, intermingle and contribute to the patient's quality of life, which in itself is also constantly changing.

Being physically cured of gynecological cancer does not necessarily mean that a patient is cured psychologically. In cases of psychological morbidity, psychotherapy may be indicated to help patients to cope more effectively and to improve the quality of their lives. Just as medical treatment is needed for a physical cure, psychological treatment may be needed for a psychological one.

REFERENCES

Abitbol, M. M. and Davenport, J. H. (1974). Sexual dysfunction after therapy for cervical cancer. *Am. J. Obstet. Gynecol.*, **119**, 181–8

American Cancer Society (1984). *Cancer Facts and Figures 1985*. American Cancer Society, New York

Amias, A. G. (1975). Sexual life after gynecological operations. *Br. Med. J.*, **ii**, 608–9

Andersen, B. L. (1984). Psychological aspects of gynaecological cancer. In Broome, A. and Wallace, L. (eds) *Psychology and Gynaecological Problems*, pp 117–41. Tavistock Publications, London

Andersen, B. L., Karlsson, J. A., Anderson, B. A. and Tewfik, H. H. (1984). Anxiety and cancer treatment: response to stressful radiotherapy. *Health Psychol.*, **3**, 535–51

Andersen, B. L. and Jochimsen, P. R. (1985). Sexual functioning among breast cancer, gynecologic cancer, and healthy women. *J. Consult. Clin. Psychol.*, **53**, 25–32

Ayres, T. (1984). Sexuality and fertility after cancer. In *Proceedings of the Fourth National Conference on Human Values and Cancer*, pp 127–33. American Cancer Society, New York

Bloom, J. A. and Ross, R. D. (1982). Measurement of the psychosocial aspects of cancer: sources of bias. In Cohen, J., Cullen, J. W. and Martin, L. R. (eds) *Psychosocial Aspects of Cancer*, pp 255–74. Raven Press, New York

Bos, G. (1984). Psychological aspects of gynaecological oncology surgery. In Heintz, A. P. M., Griffiths, C. Th. and Trimbos, J. B. (eds) *Surgery in Gynecological Oncology*, pp 307–15. Martinus Nijhoff, The Hague

Bos, G. (1986). Infertility: a price for cancer cure. In Dennerstein, L. and Fraser, I. (eds) *Proceedings of the 8th International Congress of Psychosomatic Obstetrics and Gynaecology*. Excerpta Medica, Amsterdam

Bos, G. (1986). Sexuality of gynecologic cancer patients: quantity and quality. *J. Psychosomat. Obstet. Gynecol.* (In press)

Bos, G., Rijshouwer, Y. M. and Zielstra, E. M. (1986). Quality of life of gynaecologic cancer patients: need of and possibilities for short-term psychotherapy. Internal report, Leiden

Brinkley, D. (1983). Emotional distress during cancer chemotherapy. *Br. Med. J.*, **286**, 663–4

Cain, E. N., Kohorn, E. I., Quinlan, D. M., Schwartz, P. E., Latimer, K. and Rogers, L. (1983). Psychosocial reactions to the diagnosis of gynecologic cancer. *Obstet. Gynecol.*, **62**, 635–41

Capone, M. A., Good, R. S., Westie, K. S. and Jacobson, A. F. (1980). Psychological rehabilitation of gynecologic oncology patients. *Arch. Phys. Rehabil.*, **61**, 128–32

Clark, R. L. (1976). Psychological reactions of patients and health professionals to cancer. In Cullen, J. W., Fox, B. H. and Isom, R. N. (eds) *Cancer: The Behavioral Dimensions*, pp 1–10. Raven Press, New York

Cohen, M. M. (1982). Psychosocial morbidity in cancer: a clinical perspective. In Cohen, J., Cullen, J. W. and Martin, L. R. (eds) *Psychosocial Aspects of Cancer*, pp 117–49. Raven Press, New York

Cohn, K. H. (1982). Chemotherapy from an insider's perspective. *Lancet*, **1**, 1006–9

Cullen, J. W. (1981). Research issues in psychosocial and behavioral aspects of cancer. In *Proceedings of the Third National Conference on Human Values and Cancer*, pp 157–64. American Cancer Society, New York

Danoff, B., Kramer, S., Irwin, P. and Gottlieb, A. (1983). Assessment of the quality of life in long-term survivors after definitive radiotherapy. *Am. J. Clin. Oncol. (CCT)* **6**, 339–45

Dennerstein, L., Wood, C. and Burrows, G. (1977). Sexual response following hysterectomy and oophorectomy. *Obstet. Gynecol.*, **49**, 92–6

Derogatis, L. R. (1980). Breast and gynecologic cancers. In Vaeth, J. M., Blomberg, R. C. and Adler, L. (eds) *Front. Radiat. Ther. Oncol.*, **14**, 1–11. S. Karger, Basel

Derogatis, L. R., Morrow, G. R., Fetting, J., Penman, D., Piasetsky, S., Schmale, A. M., Henrichs, M. and Carnicke, C. L. M. (1983). The prevalence of psychiatric disorders among cancer patients. *J. Am. Med. Assoc.*, **249**, 751–7

De Vita, V. T. Jr. (1982). Statement to the 13th International Cancer

Congress, Seattle. American Cancer Society, New York

Donahue, V. C. and Knapp, R. C. (1977). Sexual rehabilitation of gynecologic cancer patients. *Obstet. Gynecol.*, **49**, 118–21

Drellich, M. B., Bieber, I. and Sutherland, A. M. (1956). Adaptation to hysterectomy. In *The Psychological Impact of Cancer*, pp 88–94. American Cancer Society, New York

Dutch Society of Gynecologic Oncology (1985). Gynecologic cancer morbidity and mortality. Internal report, Leiden

Fobair, P. and Mages, N. L. (1981). Psychosocial morbidity among cancer patient survivors. In Ahmed, P. (ed.) *Living and Dying with Cancer*, pp 285–308. Elsevier, New York

Fox, B. H. (1981). Behavioral issues in cancer. In *Perspectives on Behavioral Medicine*, pp 101–33. Academic Press, New York

Golden, J. S. and Golden, M. (1980). Cancer and sex. In Vaeth, J. M., Blomberg, R. C. and Adler, L. (eds) *Front. Radiat. Ther. Oncol.*, **14**, 59–64. S. Karger, Basel

Gottesman, D. and Lewis, M. S. (1982). Differences in crises reactions among cancer and surgical patients. *J. Consult. Clin. Psychol.*, **50**, 381–8

Heintz, A. P. M. and Trimbos, J. B. (1984). New techniques for outpatient diagnosis of endometrial carcinoma. In Heintz, A. P. M., Griffiths, C. Th. and Trimbos, J. B. (eds) *Surgery in Gynecological Oncology*, pp 207–21. Martinus Nijhoff, The Hague

Hersh, P. (1982). Psychosocial aspects of patients with cancer. In De Vita, V. T., Hellman, S. and Rosenberg, S. A. (eds) *Cancer. Principles and Practice of Oncology*, pp 264–77. J. B. Lippincott Cy, Philadelphia

Holland, J. C. (1976). Coping with cancer: a challenge to the behavioral sciences. In Cullen, J. W., Fox, B. H. and Isom, R. N. (eds) *Cancer: The Behavioral Dimensions*, pp 263–8. Raven Press, New York

Holland, J. C. and Mastrovito, R. (1980). Psychologic adaptation to breast cancer. *Cancer*, **46**, 1045–52

Johnston, M. (1980). Anxiety in surgical patients. *Psychol. Med.*, **10**, 145–52

Krant, M. J. (1981). Psychosocial impact of gynecologic cancer. *Cancer*, **48**, 608–12

Lamont, J. A., De Petrillo, A. D. and Sargeant, E. J. (1978). Psychosexual rehabilitation and exenterative surgery. *Gynecol. Oncol.*, **6**, 236–42

Langer, E. J., Janis, I. V. and Wolfer, J. A. (1975). Reduction of psychological stress in surgical patients. *J. Exp. Soc. Psychol.*, **11**, 155–8

La Torre, R. A. (1978). Gender role and psychological adjustment.

Arch. Sex. Behav., **7**, 89–96

Lazarus, R. S. (1982). Stress and coping as factors in health and illness. In Cohen, J., Cullen, J. W. and Martin, L. R. (eds) *Psychosocial Aspects of Cancer*, pp 163–91. Raven Press, New York

Lennane, K. J. and Lennane, R. J. (1973). Alleged psychogenic disorders in women — possible manifestation of sexual prejudice. *New Engl. J. Med.*, **288**, 288–92

Lloyd, G. G. (1979). Psychological stress and coping mechanisms in patients with cancer. In Stoll, B. A. (ed.) *Mind and Cancer Prognosis*, pp 47–59. John Wiley & Sons Ltd, New York

Luce, J. K. (1979). Selecting patients for supportive therapy. In Stoll, B. A. (ed.) *Mind and Cancer Prognosis*, pp 127–37. John Wiley & Sons, New York

Mages, N. L., Mendelsohn, G. and Castro, J. (1980). Concepts of adaptation and life changes in cancer patients. In *Radiation Therapy, Thanatology Series*. Arno Press, New York

Maguire, G. P., Lee, E. G., Bevington, D. J., Küchemann, C. S., Crabtree, R. J. and Cornell, C. E. (1978). Psychiatric problems in the first year after mastectomy. *Br. Med. J.*, **i**, 963–5

Mantell, J. and Green, C. (1978). Reducing post-mastectomy sexual dysfunction: an appropriate role for social work. In Comfort, A. (ed.) *Sexual Consequences of Disability*, pp 207–22. Stickley Cy, Philadelphia

Mantell, J. E. (1983). The psychosocial and physiologic effects of invasive gynecologic cancers on female sexuality. In Dennerstein, L. and de Senarclens, M. (eds) *The Young Woman — Psychosomatic Aspects of Obstetrics and Gynaecology*, pp 398–408. Excerpta Medica, Amsterdam

Martin, L. R. (1982). Overview of the psychosocial aspects of cancer. In Cohen, J., Cullen, J. W. and Martin, L. R. (eds) *Psychosocial Aspects of Cancer*, pp 1–8. Raven Press, New York

Mastrovito, R. C. (1974). Cancer: awareness and denial. *Clin. Bull.*, **4**, 142–6

Morris, T., Greer, H. S. and White, P. (1977). Psychological and social adjustment to mastectomy: a two-year follow-up study. *Cancer*, **40**, 2381–7

Murphy, G. P. (1984). Progress in cancer treatment. In *Proceedings of the Fourth National Conference on Human Values and Cancer*, pp 2–6. American Cancer Society, New York

Newell, G. R., Boutwell, W. B., Morris, D. L., Tilley, B. C. and Branyon, E. S. (1982). Epidemiology of cancer. In De Vita, V. T., Hellman, S. and Rosenberg, S. A. (eds) *Cancer. Principles and Practice of*

Oncology, pp 3–22. J. B. Lippincott Cy, Philadelphia

Peck, A. (1972). Emotional reactions to having had cancer. *Am. J. Roentgenol. Radium Ther. Nucl. Med.*, **144**, 591–9

Peck, A. and Boland, J. (1977). Emotional reactions to radiation treatment. *Cancer*, **40**, 180–4

Perez, C. A., Knapp, R. C. and Young, R. C. (1982). Gynecologic tumors. In De Vita, V. T., Hellman, S. and Rosenberg, S. A. (eds) *Cancer. Principles and Practice of Oncology*, pp 823–83. J. B. Lippincott Cy, Philadelphia

Reading, A. E. (1981). Psychological preparation for surgery: patient recall of information. *J. Psychosomat. Res.*, **25**, 57–62

Schain, W. S. (1981). Role of the sex therapist in the care of the cancer patient. In Vaeth, J. M., Blomberg, R. C. and Adler, L. (eds) *Front. Radiat. Ther. Oncol.*, **15**, 168–83. S. Karger, Basel

Sewell, H. H. and Edwards, D. W. (1980). Pelvic genital cancer: body image and sexuality. In Vaeth, J. M., Blomberg, R. C. and Adler, L. (eds) *Front. Radiat. Ther. Oncol.*, **14**, 35–41. S. Karger, Basel

Silberfarb, P. M., Philibert, D. and Levine, P. M. (1980). Psychosocial aspects of neoplastic disease: II. Affective and cognitive effects of chemotherapy in cancer patients. *Am. J. Psychiat.*, **137**, 597–601

Sime, A. M. (1976). Relationship of preoperative fear, type of coping and information received about surgery and recovery from surgery. *J. Personal. Soc. Psychol.*, **34**, 716–9

Small, E. Ch., Anderson, B., Watring, W. G., Edinger, D. D. and Mitchell, G. W. (1983). Ovarian carcinoma: management of stress in patients and physicians. *Gynecol. Oncol.*, **15**, 160–5

Sontag, S. (1979). *Illness as Metaphor*. A. Lane, London

Spinetta, J. J. (1981). Problems in evaluation of psychosocial research. In *Proceedings of the Third National Conference on Human Values and Cancer*, pp 151–7. American Cancer Society, New York

Sutherland, A. M. and Orbach, C. E. (1953). Depressive reactions associated with surgery for cancer. In *The Psychological Impact of Cancer*, pp 17–21. American Cancer Society, New York (1977)

Trimbos, J. B. (1985). The management of ovarian cancer stage I–IIA. In *Current Concepts in Gynecological Oncology*, pp 151–4. Boerhaave Committee for Postgraduate Medical Education, Noordwijkerhout

Vettese, J. M. (1976). Problems of the patients confronting the diagnosis of cancer. In Cullen, J. W., Fox, B. H. and Isom, R. N. (eds) *Cancer: the Behavioral Dimensions*, pp 275–82. Raven Press, New York

Vincent, C. E., Vincent, B., Greiss, F. C. and Linton, E. B. (1975).

Some marital-sexual concomitants of carcinoma of the cervix. *Southern Med. J.*, **68**, 552–8

Weideger, P. (1976). *Menstruation and Menopause*. Knopf, New York

Weisman, A. D. and Worden, J. W. (1976–77). The existential plight in cancer: significance of the first 100 days. *Int. J. Psychiat. Med.*, **7**, 1–15

Wallace, L. (1984). Psychological preparation for gynaecological surgery. In Broome, A. and Wallace, L. (eds) *Psychology and Gynaecological Problems*, pp 161–88. Tavistock Publications, London

Index

alcohol and drug abuse, 42

cancer, gynecological, 167–84
  physical effects of surgery, 168–70
  psychological effects, 169, 170–1
  reactions of patients to
    breast surgery, 175–6
    chemotherapy, 177–8
    diagnosis, 167–8, 172–5
    medical treatments, 175
    radiotherapy, 176–7
  socio-cultural effects, 169, 171–2
  survivors, quality of life in, 178–84
    long-term, 180–2
    research project Leiden, 182–3
    short-term, 179–80
chronic pelvic pain, 105–17
  management of, 114–16
  organic causes of, 106–10
  psychological causes of, 110–13
confidentiality, 13
contraception
  acceptability factors, 57–68
    intrapersonal, 61–3
    physical, 64
    sexual, 63
    socio-cultural, 58–61
  adverse side-effects, 67–8
  effects on sexual behaviour, 64–8
  in history, 55–6
  reasons for, 56–7
coping strategies, 16–17
counselling
  of infertile patients, 100–2
  of patients requesting reversal of tubal ligation, 148
crisis-intervention, 31–2

doctor-patient relationship, 11–18, 97–9

Government attitudes towards contraception, 58
gynecologist
  and contraception, 64, 68
  and hysterectomy, 124–5
  qualities of, 12–14
  role of, 14–18, 33–4

hypnosis, 32–3
hysterectomy, 119–35
  clinical management of patients, 132–5
  depression following, 134–5
  frequency of, 120–5
  in history, 119–20
  psychological and sexual sequelae, 125–32

infertility, 87–102
  clinical management of patients, 97–102
  female, 91
  investigations of, 89–90
  in-vitro fertilization, 95–7
  male, 91–2
  reactions to, 88–9
  unexplained, 92–5
interviewing of patients or couples, 14–18, 47–50, 99–100, 132–3, 134, 148, 162
intrapsychic conflict, 46

investigations, clinical or laboratory, 18, 50, 89–90, 114–15, 162
in-vitro fertilization, 95–7

learned sexual dysfunction, causes of
  family attitudes, 44–6
  religious orthodoxy, 46

marital therapy, 30–1
medications, effect of on sexual behaviour, 43, 68
menopause, 151–63
  behavioural changes in, 153–61
    biological causes of, 154–7
    psychological causes of, 157–8
    sociological causes of, 158–61
  clinical management of patients, 161–3
  definition of, 151
  psychological complaints, 152
  sexual complaints, 153
menstruation
  affective variations during cycle, 73–4
  premenstrual tension syndrome, 75–85
  psychiatric disorders and, 74

oral contraceptive pill
  adverse side-effects of, 56, 64, 67–8, 79
  beneficial side-effects of, 79
  effectiveness of, 57
  effect of on sexual behaviour, 65–7, 68

physical examination, 18, 49–50
  for infertility, 89–90
premenstrual tension syndrome, 75–85
  causes of, 77–82
  clinical management of patients, 82–5
  definition of, 75
  methodological problems, 75–7
psychosexual dysfunction, 37–46
  assessment of, 46–50
  intrapsychic, 46
  learned, 44–6
  management of, 50–3
  symptomatic, 40–4

types of, 38–9
psychosomatic, meaning of, 9–11
psychotherapy, 21–30
  behavioural, 27–30
  long-term, 24–26
  psychoanalysis, 24
  supportive, 26–7

religion, 46, 145
  and contraception, 59–61

sexual changes due to age, 36
sexual problems, 35–53
  management of, 50–3
  psychosexual dysfunction, 37–50
  unrealistic expectations, 36
sterilization, tubal, 139–48
  adverse sequelae to, 140–1, 146–7
  clinical management, 146–8
  request for reversal of, 143–5
  sexual adjustment to, 142
surgery, effect of on sexual behaviour, 43–4
symptomatic sexual dysfunction, causes of
  alcohol and drug abuse, 42
  iatrogenic, 42–4
  interpersonal, 40
  organic, 40–1
  psychiatric, 41–4

therapy techniques
  crisis-intervention, 31–2
  for chronic pelvic pain, 115–16
  for menopausal complaints, 162–3
  for post-hysterectomy depression, 134–5
  for premenstrual tension, 84–5
  for sexual dysfunctions, 52–3
  hormone, 78–81, 84, 133–4, 154–7, 162–3
  hypnosis, 32–3
  marital, 30–1
  psychotherapy, 21–30